Erotic
Aromatherapy

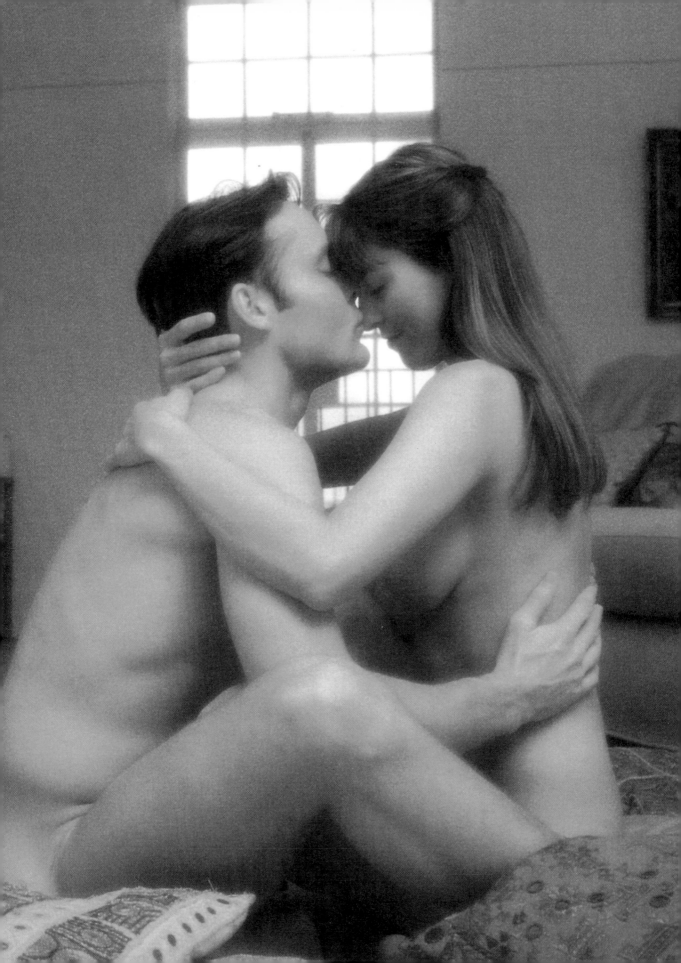

Erotic Aromatherapy
Essential Oils for Lovers

CHRISSIE WILDWOOD

PHOTOGRAPHY BY DALE DURFEE
AND STEPHEN MARWOOD

Sterling Publishing Co., Inc. New York

To Howard, with love

PLEASE NOTE
The author, publisher and packager cannot accept responsibility for
misadventure resulting from the use of essential oils, or any other
therapeutic methods that are mentioned in this book.

Published 1994 by Sterling Publishing Company, Inc.
387 Park Avenue South, New York, N.Y. 10016
Originally published 1994 in Great Britain
by Headline Book Publishing, a division of Hodder Headline PLC
338 Euston Road, London NW1 3BH under the title *Sensual Aromatherapy*
Text copyright © Chrissie Wildwood 1994
Photographs copyright © Dale Durfee and Stephen Marwood 1994
This edition copyright © Eddison Sadd Editions 1994
Distributed in Canada by Sterling Publishing
c/o Canadian Manda Group, P.O. Box 920, Station U
Toronto, Ontario, Canada M8Z 5P9

Library of Congress Cataloging-in-Publication Data Available

2 4 6 8 10 9 7 5 3 1

AN EDDISON·SADD EDITION
Edited, designed and produced by
Eddison Sadd Editions Limited
St Chad's Court, 146B King's Cross Road
London WC1X 9DH

Phototypeset in Cochin using QuarkXPress on Apple Macintosh
Origination by Tipongraph S.r.l., Italy
Printed and bound by Graficromo, S.A., Cordoba, Spain

Sterling ISBN 0-8069-0736-3

Contents

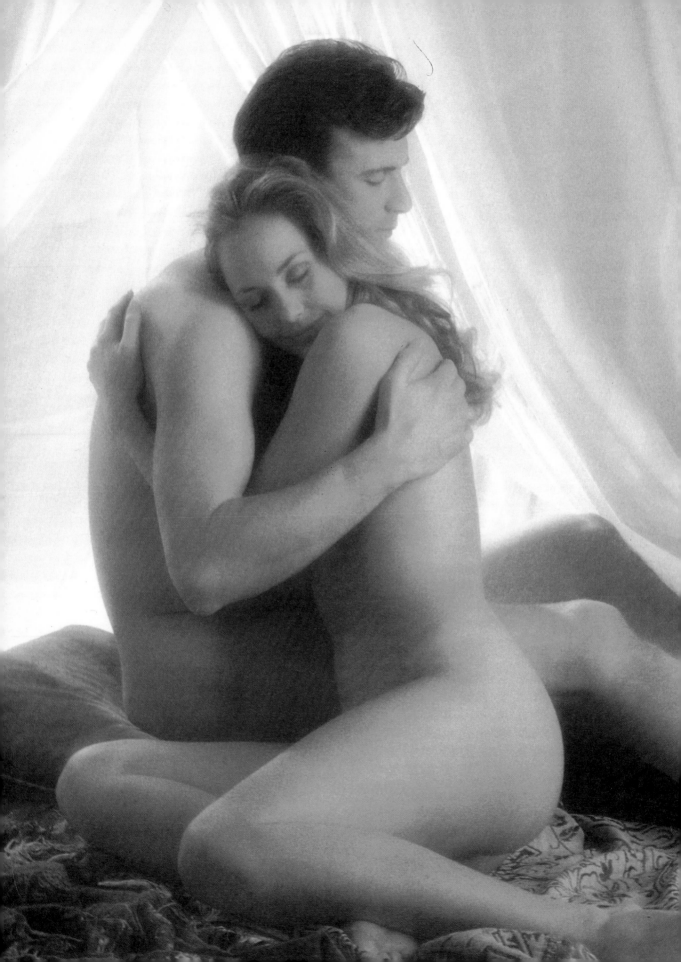

Introduction

*Yes, it's true the senses can lead you astray
and the pursuit of pleasure can get you in trouble.
Sensual pleasure needs the guidance of
practical and ethical judgement. But you won't gain
good health by repeatedly vetoing the vote
of the senses and denigrating the wisdom of the body.
Nature was neither capricious nor perverted
in making sure that, other things being equal,
what feels good is good for you.*

George Leonard

Imagine spending many timeless moments indulging the senses with your lover, exploring beautiful sounds, sights, tastes, textures and scents – and the body and soul of your beloved. To imagine is the first step; to put it into practice is the next. In so doing, you may happen upon the key to the temple of Aphrodite. And in the presence of the goddess of beauty and love, you may transcend the boundary of the senses to experience ecstasy.

'Oh come on now – ecstasy? We are far too familiar with each other to recapture anything like that.' If this cynical remark mirrors your own feelings about the quality of your relationship, then this book was written for you. True, it is easy to feel bored with sex in a long-term relationship and find yourself wishing that you could rekindle the flames of passion. Embarking on a potentially disastrous love affair is not the answer. Emotional upheavals apart, in the age of AIDS and other sexually transmitted diseases, we owe it to ourselves, our partners and the children we have or may conceive, to play safe. However, as you are about to discover, safe sex with a familiar partner need not be boring – especially when enhanced by delicious fragrances and bonded with love. The art of sensuous aromatherapy, which explores the sensual, uplifting and healing properties of nature's aromatic essences, will add an ambience of enchantment to your love life.

Although we shall explore the erotic and therapeutic properties of essential oils in subsequent chapters, suffice it to say here that aromatherapy has at last emerged from the wings of relative obscurity into the limelight of popular awareness. Just why it should have captured the imagination on such a grand scale is not too difficult to understand. Apart from the remarkable healing properties of essential oils, this beautiful healing art is creative. For much of the skill of the aromatherapist (or the adventurous essential oil user) lies in their ability to concoct wonderful mood-enhancing, pleasure-inspiring fragrances.

Unlike more clinical therapies, such as homoeopathy or acupuncture, aromatherapy can also be fun! This is why it lends itself most readily to love play. It combines massage with scent, thus awakening our most primitive, yet most highly evolved senses: smell and touch. Add music and a pleasing setting and we also nurture our auditory and visual senses.

It is my own belief that a fulfilling and loving relationship (which may or may not involve sexual intercourse) is the most potent healing force in the universe. In fact, researchers have demonstrated that positive emotions, especially the giving and receiving of love, act to strengthen our immune defences. Unhappiness, on the other hand, lowers our resistance to all manner of physical ills – be it colds, flu, shingles or something much more serious. We also know that people can truly die of a broken heart – such is the power of emotion.

Although the emphasis of this book is on aromatherapy for lovers, space is also given to the all-important concept of self-love. Before we can truly love another, we must first love ourselves. We might 'need' someone, cling to them, pity them, idealize them – but only when our own cup is full to the brim can it overflow to others. Indeed, positive self-esteem is the foundation for enjoying life and creating healthy relationships. Yet many people believe that they would love themselves if only someone would love them first. As psychologist Margo Annand puts it: 'You are the principal source of your pleasure. Instead of looking outside for the right partner, you give to yourself first everything that you would give to your beloved'.

However, loving yourself in this way does not mean being narcissistic and disregarding of others. Rather, it means regarding yourself as a person worthy of the love and respect that you would feel for a good friend.

One way of honouring the 'inner lover' is to make full use of the mood-enhancing effects of nature's essential oils. As this book shows, they can be used in a variety of ways to nurture our self-esteem. For instance, they can be used in the bath, or vaporized in the home to create a special ambience, or perhaps made into a luxurious body oil.

'This is all very well, but we don't have enough time, or even the privacy to spend many hours pampering ourselves or caressing each other with aromatic oils.'

Every parent will commiserate with such a lament. Moreover, looking after children all day can be even more taxing than going out to work. The lack of mental stimulus, and the absence of social contact may lead to discontentment and depression, which can quell the flames of desire. However, it is possible to steal some quality time to be alone with your partner if you really want to. Although it may mean a juggling act, the reward will be worth far more than the effort expended. As well as heightening intimacy and enhancing your mood, these qualities are bound to positively affect others in your sphere, especially children. As children are so receptive to the changes in mood of their parents, they will respond by becoming more joyful and relaxed themselves.

Incidentally, it is worth mentioning in passing that traditional massage (with or without essential oils) can be enjoyed by the whole family. In parts of India where massage is virtually a way of life, the skill has been handed down from parent to child for centuries. Gentle stroking, especially of the feet, is soothing and balancing to the hyperactive child or fractious baby. If you would like to know more about traditional aromatherapy and massage, see the Bibliography on page 156 for a list of excellent books on the subject.

Using this book, you can select ideas to enhance any stolen moment with your partner. If you are a parent, do try to enlist the help of family and friends, perhaps building a supportive baby-sitting network, so that you and your partner can take those stolen moments. Sharing the responsibility for minding the children provides you with the opportunity to spend some time alone together. Parents of older children may even manage an afternoon of lovemaking while the children are at school. It may mean taking a day off work, but what better way to use up your holiday entitlement? Or better still, you may even snatch the odd weekend away – taking your precious oils with you, of course.

Before we go any further, it should be stressed that this book is not about the 'nuts and bolts' of sexual technique – inventive positions, pin-pointing the G-spot, and such like. There are many books on this subject. Rather, this book is about the use of tender loving touch and other sensory joys as a means to awaken the spirit of playfulness and spontaneity in a loving relationship; joys which too many adults leave behind in childhood. It is also about relaxation and self-acceptance.

Even though the images in this book depict heterosexual love in the guise of youth and physical beauty – that is to say, beauty in the eyes of the Western beholder – please accept this as poetic licence. In reality, love knows no such bounds. Sensual aromatherapy is for lovers of all shapes and sizes, irrespective of age and sexual orientation. It is also for those wishing to enhance their love-life through the alchemy of fragrance and the magic of touch. Have fun!

Chrissie Wildwood

Chrissie Wildwood, February 1994

Before You Begin

When using essential oils for the first time, especially if you have sensitive skin, it is best to pre-test the diluted essence (or blend of essences) beforehand. Rub a little behind the ears (a supersensitive spot) and leave for 24 hours. If there is no redness or itching, the oil is safe for you to use.

It is also important to point out that the perfume strength blends suggested in this book may not be suitable for those with sensitive skin. Essential oils intended for massage are usually diluted at the rate of 1 or 2 drops to every teaspoon of a vegetable oil base such as almond or sunflower oil. However, the quantity of essential oil in perfume blends is much higher than this (6 to 10 drops to 1 teaspoon of base oil). Therefore if you have sensitive skin or know you have an allergy to commercial perfume, you may also have to forego the use of natural skin perfumes. However, you could enjoy room scents instead, or perhaps perfume your clothes (outer garments only) or the ends of your hair.

Never use an oil about which you can find little or no information. Unfortunately, there are a number of potentially hazardous oils readily available to the public. Oils such as aniseed, balsam of Peru, elecampane (also known as inula), hyssop, tarragon, winter savory, summer savory, thyme and sage (not to be confused with clary sage which is safe to use) are best avoided by the layperson as they are very powerful. However, all the oils featured in this book are safe to use if they are correctly diluted as specified.

Pregnancy

A number of oils stimulate menstruation and therefore the aromatherapy associations advise against pregnant women using such oils, especially in the first three months of pregnancy when miscarriage is more of a threat than later

on. Other potentially hazardous oils are those containing stimulating substances which have a strong effect on the nervous system. In reality, however, one would need to apply (or take by mouth) a very high concentration of these risky essences to cause miscarriage. Nevertheless, it is always best to err on the side of caution. Before using any essential oil, please check that it is safe for you to do so. Refer to the aromatic profiles (*see Chapter 3*). Where appropriate, a CAUTIONS note is included at the end of specific profile. It is also advisable to use *all* essential oils in the lowest recommended concentration at this time. Avoid using skin perfume-strength blends.

Nursing Mothers

It is advisable to avoid the use of perfume-strength blends directly on the skin while breastfeeding. Due to their tiny molecular structure, plant essences (and some synthetic perfume chemicals) can slip through the skin and find their way into the bloodstream and other body fluids. Many can also cross the placental barrier. Although there is no hard evidence to suggest that mothers and babies have been harmed by perfumes, I still feel it is best to err on the side of caution. Moreover, some essential oils can be very stimulating to young babies, especially geranium essence, and may interfere with natural sleep patterns.

Falsification of Melissa Oil

True melissa oil is extremely difficult to obtain as so little is produced. When it is available, the oil is as costly as rose otto. Most of the so-called melissa oils on the market are blends of infinitely cheaper essences such as lemongrass, lemon and citronella. Therefore, rather than be hoodwinked by unscrupulous suppliers, it is best to avoid this oil. Only when you have smelled true melissa essence and compared it to the falsified versions will you be better able to tell the difference. For these obvious reasons, melissa does not feature in this book.

Amber

If you come across this oil, be suspicious. It is certain to be a synthetic compound or a blend of clary sage and benzoin (a vanilla-like resinoid). As far as I am aware, true amber essence, from the fossilized resin, is unobtainable. Ambergris (a substance excreted from the sperm whale, sometimes found floating on the sea) is also known as 'amber', an extremely costly fragrance material used in high-class perfumes. Ambergris is not generally available to the public.

Essential Oils and the Breasts

There are a number of aromatherapists who claim that phytohormones (plant hormones) can be used to increase breast size. Just because there are oils which stimulate milk flow in nursing mothers, it does not mean that they can be used to enlarge the breasts of women who are not breastfeeding. It is extremely doubtful that oils such as anise, fennel, caraway and lemongrass have any effect on breast size one way or the other and to claim otherwise is misleading.

One aromatherapy author even suggests oils to diminish breast size! Jojoba oil is recommended as a base 'because of its emulsifying properties' and rose essence 'because it is an astringent'. The mind boggles. Such ludicrous claims do nothing for the reputation of respectable aromatherapy.

Quality Control

A pure essential oil is one which has been produced from a named botanical source (for example, lavender, *Lavandula angustifolia*), and has not been extended or modified with synthetic substances or other essential oils. Essential oil suppliers have established a form of certification known as AROMARK Grade for essential oils that can be guaranteed natural. In India, the government has given the term AGMARK (Agricultural Guarantee Mark) to some of their oils, mainly sandalwood and lemongrass. Any oil carrying the AROMARK or AGMARK signature is guaranteed to be a pure unadulterated plant essence. (*For further information on buying essential oils, see page 52.*)

General Cautions

- Keep bottles out of reach of children.
- Do not apply neat oils directly to the skin as they can cause irritation.
- Keep oils away from the eyes, and do not rub your eyes after handling them. Should any essential oil get into your eyes, rinse it out with plenty of fresh water; seek medical advice if necessary.
- Never take essential oils by mouth, unless under medical instructions.
- Some homoeopaths believe that all essential oils weaken or cancel out the effects of homoeopathic remedies. Other practitioners believe that only the camphoraceous oils are contra-indicated, for example, camphor, eucalyptus, peppermint and rosemary. If in doubt, check with your homoeopathic practitioner beforehand.

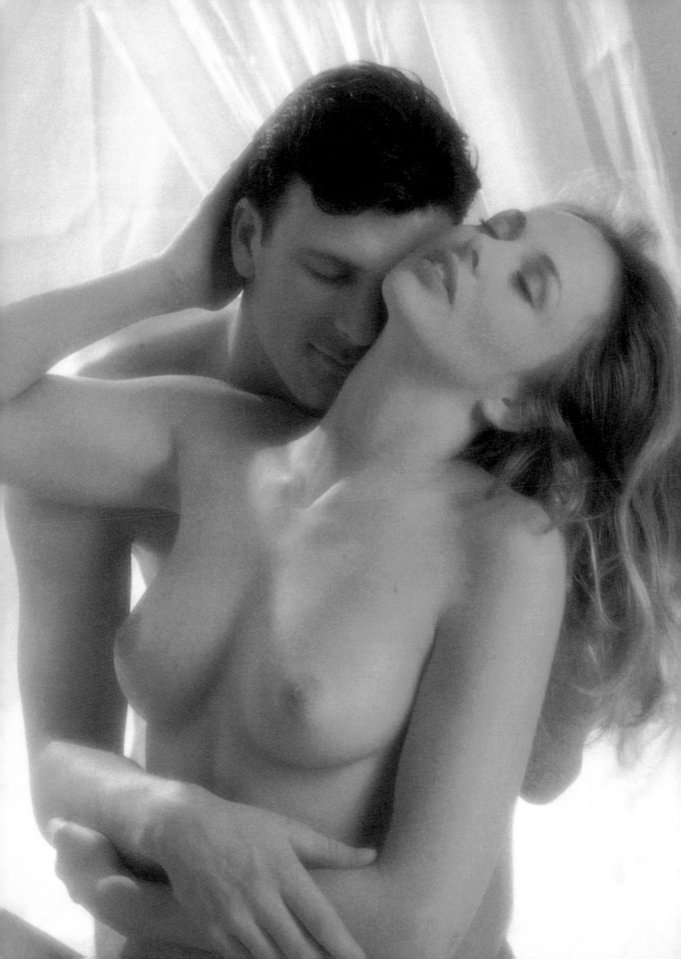

CHAPTER 1

The Enigmatic Sense

*In a world sayable and lush, where marvels offer
themselves up readily for verbal dissection,
smells are often right on the tip of our tongues – but no
closer – and it gives them a kind of magical distance,
a mystery, a power without a name,
a sacredness.*

Diane Ackerman

Scent of the Past

A mere whiff of a certain fragrance is enough to transport you swiftly through the labyrinth of mind to a timeless dimension of memories, images and feelings. A place where you recapture the joy of first love, perhaps, when the days were adorned with laughter; the nights, blue velvet and silver. Another scent may recall a half-forgotten walk in the misty wildwood; a third, fond memories of a well-loved grandmother. And curiously, a scent may trigger the frustrated response: 'It reminds me of something, but I can't think what'.

Yet there is no short-term memory with odour; what you encounter can be recalled over and over again. But just as a fragrance may summon to mind a joyful memory, another may cause the heart to move with grief. Because of the strength of this evocative power, it is perhaps best to let your lover smell any oils you plan to use, to ensure that those you have chosen do not have unhappy associations.

Then there are those scents which evoke a certain feeling for no apparent reason, and the effect may be generalized. That is to say, other people may experience a similar response to the odour. A friend of mine finds the blunt scent of chrysanthemums melancholic. It seems D. H. Lawrence did too, as reflected in the title of his short story *Odour of Chrysanthemums*, a depressing tale set in a mining village. Similarly, many people perceive as solemn the aromatic oils of cypress and violet leaf. But aromatherapists have discovered that such fragrances can be soothing to people suffering from anxious states of mind. Cypress is especially beneficial in this respect, for its cooling scent engenders a sense of quietude.

Experience has also shown that the essences of citrus fruits smell cheerful to most people. The essential oil of bergamot, obtained from a small orange-like fruit, is especially popular. As well as being the principal ingredient of uplifting eau-de-cologne formulas, it is used to flavour Earl Grey tea.

However, the most fascinating aromatics of all must surely be those that have been used for centuries in the art of allurement, as charms and love potions. In fact, the essences of flowers, roots and woods such as rose, jasmine, ylang ylang, vetiver and sandalwood are still employed by the modern weaver of enchantment – the perfumier – to stir the imagination and to awaken sensuality. Whether these sweet-smelling elixirs really can work such magic we shall explore later. Suffice to say that studies have shown that many aromatic plants exude enticing substances with a similar chemical make-up to that of our own sexual secretions. But this is not the whole story. Unlike animals, people react to perfumes in a great number of sophisticated, emotionally complex and imaginative ways.

As Kipling said: 'Smells are surer than sights and sounds to make your heart strings crack'. Indeed, it is virtually impossible to smell anything without an emotional response – whether it be a simple like/dislike reaction, or something much more complex. This is because the basic instinct of smell bypasses the logical thought processes concerned with language. Try describing a particular odour to someone who has not smelled it before and you will know what I mean. At best, it can only be defined by another odour or another sense, including the 'sixth sense' as reflected in what is commonly known as the 'spirit of place'. For instance, a perfume may smell sweetly mellow with a hint of vanilla, or cool and green with a sharp edge or, more imaginatively, raucous like a scarlet-clad trumpet player, or dark and mysterious like the damp forest floor.

Imaginative forays aside, just how are odours perceived, and why do they have such a profound influence on mood?

The Effects of Odours

Before the microscopic airborne particles of an odoriferous substance can be detected, they must be drawn up with the in-breath to a yellow-brown patch in the roof of the nose. This is the olfactory *epithelium*, measuring about five centimetres square, containing up to 50 million odour receptor cells bearing minuscule hair-like structures called *cilia*. These cells are specialized sensory neurones (technically speaking they are brain cells) embedded in a mucous membrane, each of which connects directly with the brain by means of a single long nerve fibre. Unlike ordinary brain cells which cannot be replaced once destroyed, the sensitive olfactory cells are in a constant state of decline and regeneration, thus indicating their importance to our basic needs.

Once in contact with the olfactory epithelium, the odour molecules are dissolved in the mucus. Responses to the molecules (not the odour molecules themselves) are then sent up to the brain in the form of electrochemical impulses via the nerve fibres to the olfactory bulb – a part of the brain which actually extends into the nose. The odour molecules, having triggered their effect, eventually disconnect from the receptor cells and float away on the out-breath.

Smell impulses, unlike the signals of the other senses, bypass the part of the brain that gives rise to our intellect – the neocortex – and go directly to the behaviour centres, the limbic system or 'smell brain'. Although this area is still largely uncharted territory, we do know that it is concerned with our instinctive drives: emotion, intuition, memory, creativity, hunger, thirst, sleep patterns, sex drive and probably much else besides.

From this, it is easier to understand how odours influence both the physical and emotional aspects of our being. To take a simple and well-known example: the delicious aroma of your favourite food will stimulate your appetite by making your mouth water and at the same time cause the digestive juices in the stomach to flow. If it is a special festive dish, you will more than likely have many joyful memories to savour as well.

Altered States

Moreover, the phenomena associated with altered states of consciousness also arise from the limbic system: out of body sensations, visions of white or golden light, feelings of euphoria – experiences known to those practising advanced methods of meditation, or as a result of taking certain drugs. So from what we have already learned about the sense of smell, the ancient idea that incense and perfume elevates the human spirit to other dimensions of awareness is not as naïve or as far-fetched as it once may have seemed.

As a matter of interest, scientists in Germany have recently discovered that frankincense resin contains the psychoactive substance trahydrocannabinole, which is released when the resin is burned as incense. Frankincense is still burned in Catholic churches; but I wonder how many priests and churchgoers are aware of its hidden depths? It would seem that frankincense is much more than a psychological prop, a mere symbol of religious mysticism. It is actually a material trigger, albeit a subtle one, acting to blur the edges of concrete reality, thus predisposing the individual to certain meditative states of mind.

In apparent contradiction to the 'holy smoke' explanation, Australian scientist Dr Michael Stoddard found something else in frankincense (and also in myrrh): substances akin to male and female sex hormones. According to Stoddard, the ancients used such aromatics to awaken sexual, ecstatic energies. However, the aim may have been to transmute sexual energy into 'higher' states of awareness. In fact, 'mystical hedonism' – a technique employing the full use of the senses to overcome the senses, or to attain spiritual transformation – is still used in certain Eastern religious traditions.

So, if the aroma is liked, the preparatory function of frankincense (and other aromatics) can be employed for erotic and/or spiritual purposes. It is entirely a matter of focus. The mind, however, remains in the driving seat – even when subjected to infinitely more powerful mood-altering substances.

Indeed, it is a well-known fact that hospice patients with untreatable cancers who also experience distressing emotions such as fear, depression or a sense of isolation, often require high doses of morphine (derived from the opium poppy) to control their pain. The same patients, having learned to accept their condition with the help of specialized counselling and the close support of their loved ones – and in some enlightened hospices, gentle aromatherapy massage – often find their need for morphine markedly reduced. In the right circumstances, the body produces its own natural opiates, or 'happiness substances', in the form of endorphins, enkephalins and the mood-altering chemical phenylethylamine (PEA).

Interestingly, PEA is released by the body in response to all life's pleasures: smelling lovely fragrances, eating delicious food, receiving nurturing massage, falling in love, listening to uplifting music, being moved by a beautiful scene, and so on. PEA is also found in certain foods, most notably chocolate and cheese; its chemical sister phenylethylalcohol is a constituent of rosewater.

Smell Range

Although there are considerable differences between the smell sensitivities of individuals, generally speaking the healthy human nose can detect over 10,000 different odours. Perfumiers and native hunters, however, may be able to detect several times as many odours, both in higher dilution and from a greater distance. This is because the sense of smell can be enhanced through training. In which case this must surely dispel the myth that the human olfactory sense has diminished as a result of evolution.

While a super-efficient sense of smell is no longer vital to our existence, when circumstances arise to make it so, then a different pattern emerges. One famous person with a highly developed sense of smell was the American Helen Keller, who was deprived of all her senses, excepting touch and smell. She could identify friends and visitors by their personal odours. And simply by smelling people she said that she could decipher 'the work they are engaged in. The odours of the wood, iron, paint and drugs cling to the garments of those who work in them ... When a person passes quickly from one place to another, I get a scent impression of where he has been – the kitchen, the garden, or the sickroom'. However, even the most highly developed olfactory sense tires when subjected to the same odour for even a short while. The olfactory cells become 'saturated' or tired, and cease to detect the odour, though there may be a fleeting reminder of its presence from time to time. Nevertheless, you may have discovered that a detested odour will seem to linger for an eternity. Clearly, there is a powerful auto-suggestive element to smell. Indeed, if we adore (or dislike) an odour intensely enough we can apparently conjure up its presence from nothing.

Some years ago as a new student of aromatherapy at my first workshop, I encountered the captivating aroma of sandalwood. I put the bottle down, but later, because I was so enchanted with its dulcet tones of aroma, I decided to go back for another whiff. Yes, it was truly divine. But as I replaced the cap, to my amazement, I noticed it was labelled 'Geranium' – I had picked up the wrong bottle.

Anyone familiar with the clear, intensely sweet aroma of geranium essence would know that one would need to be totally smell-warped to confuse it with the soft, deep notes of sandalwood. Needless to say, as soon as I realized my error, the spell had been broken; the scent of geranium came through shrill and clear.

Never since have I been able to work such magic – at least not on myself. Strictly for research purposes, however, I have succeeded in hoodwinking others into believing that a disliked essence was present in a blend of aromatic oils. (It is actually more difficult to convince people of the opposite.) Having discovered the dupe, one person in particular became most irate with disbelief – he was certain that the 'horrible' lavender had actually been present, and that the experiment itself was some kind of double bluff!

Anosmia

Sadly, there are those people who cannot smell anything at all; they suffer from anosmia. Others may lack sensitivity for specific odours, particularly to some musks; they are partially anosmic. Similarly, it is common to have selected odour blindness to the aroma of sandalwood, which is possessed of a musky element. However, when the musky (some would say 'urinous') note can be detected, it is either adored or detested. Then there are those who are only aware of the soft, woody overtone of the fragrance.

Indeed, odours are multifaceted; a single odoriferous material may be composed of many different overtones and undertones. Just why an individual should perceive only an aspect of a particular aroma, or indeed why we should like some fragrances and not others, is still something of a mystery. However, from an aromatherapy perspective, it is known that we are drawn to those aromas which are right for our needs at a given time. As our emotional and physical state alters, so may our aroma preferences change.

Although it is possible to be born without a sense of smell, anosmia is more often associated with nutritional deficiencies, allergy, nasal polyps, ageing, a brain tumour or exposure to toxic chemicals. Whatever the cause, life without a sense of smell is often accompanied by a depressed outlook. And quite apart from the dangers of being unable to detect the odours of something burning, gas leaks or spoiled food, the condition renders the most ambrosial food tasteless. Most of us have experienced this when suffering from a heavy cold. This is because smell and taste are interrelated functions. It has also been reported that a quarter of sufferers of anosmia experience loss of libido – but not every sufferer. Loss of libido as a result of anosmia may be also related to the associated depression which accompanies the condition (depression is a well-known dampener of sexual desire), and not just because the person can no longer smell their partner's sexual secretions.

While the human ear may be 'deaf' to high and low frequency sound, as every physicist knows, this does not mean that we cannot be affected by them. Likewise, we can respond both physically and emotionally to low level fragrance. Researchers at Warwick University (England), 'wired up' a number of volunteers to an EEG (electroencephalograph) instrument which records the electrical activity of the brain and skin. When exposed to fragrance so highly diluted as to be totally imperceptible to the subjects, very clear skin responses were recorded. Moreover, activity in the olfactory area of the brain was evident. It appears that the skin and brain simultaneously respond to the subtle effects of odour.

Clearly, we humans are far more sensitive to the environment than we realize. It could be argued that sufferers of anosmia may benefit, albeit on a subliminal level, from the scent of honeysuckle in the air, or from aromatherapy treatment or perfume.

Natural Body Scent and Pheromones

People, as well as plants, insects and animals, secrete subtly fragrant hormone-like chemicals called pheromones. The word 'pheromone' was coined by researchers in 1959 and is derived from the Greek *pherin*, to transfer, and *hormone*, to excite. Hormones are internal messengers. They are secreted into the bloodstream to influence the activity of target cells. The closely-related pheromones are external messengers; they are radiated by the skin to evoke a response in other people.

Some pheromones play a part in sexual attraction, while others contribute to our characteristic body scent. There are also those pheromones which communicate the odour of emotion. Unlike most animals, which are very conscious of the odour nuances of mood, most humans perceive these odours on a subliminal level. Nevertheless, the odour of emotion can have a powerful and immediate effect on those nearby. As researchers into crowd behaviour would confirm, intense emotions such as fear, joy, anger and despair can spread like wildfire. Think of an excited football crowd.

While no two people smell exactly alike, there are similarities between races. There are also recognizable 'male' and 'female' odours to be found within any ethnic group. Body scent is also determined by the type of food eaten, the odours of which appear in our bodily fluids, most noticeably in sweat. In a healthy person, the odorants in fresh sweat are not at all offensive. It is only when the resident skin bacteria start to break it down, producing an excess of lactic acid, that it becomes malodorant.

However, nothing can alter the underlying 'fingerprint' odour – that which reflects the unique essence of our being. If this were not so, a dog would fail to recognize its owner should the person suddenly indulge in a vindaloo or douse themselves with perfume.

The 'fingerprint' odour apart, illness, the pill (and other drugs), as well as hormonal changes such as puberty, pregnancy, menstruation and the menopause also influence our body odour. Moreover, our body odour influences our choice of perfume. When the perfume is applied to the skin, it intermingles with our own body chemistry. This explains why the same perfume smells different on each person, and why we tend to go off certain perfumes (and flavours) from time to time and begin to enjoy those previously distasteful to us.

The Scents of Desire

To discuss human sexuality in terms of pheromones can be something of a 'turn off'. After all, there must be more to love than the musky odour of androstenone. Indeed, unlike animals whose sexual cycles are governed by the release of pheromones, we humans are more highly evolved. The prefrontal lobe of the brain, which is absent in animals, acts to filter instinct. This means we can maintain a measure of control over our 'animal' desires.

However, just like a flower whose fragrance declares to the world that it is both fertile and desirable, during sexual excitement we humans produce a cascade of enticing scent molecules. They are found in the milky fluid produced by the aprocrine system – a collection of specialized sweat glands found primarily in the armpits, pubic area, face and nipples. Hair, especially axillary and pubic hair, facilitates the radiation of these sexual odours. Pheromones are also found in the vaginal secretions, semen and saliva. During sexual arousal the apocrine glands in the face are especially active, which is part of the reason why kissing is so enjoyable.

Of the 200 separate components distinguishable in normal body odours, the musky androstenone is the principal chemical of attraction. It is a biochemical cousin of the male sex hormone testosterone, which is produced in the female body too – albeit in minuscule quantities. Similarly, a tiny amount of the female hormone oestrogen is produced in the male body. Testosterone and androstenone comprise the 'raw fuel' of the libido in both sexes. Androstenone in particular is believed to play a major role in regulating the menstrual cycle. Indeed, frequent lovemaking with a male partner, which serves to transfer appreciable amounts of the pheromone, can promote regular menstruation in a woman whose cycle is jerky. Males experience an androstenone peak during their thirties, but its presence slowly diminishes as they age. However, the pheromone virtually ceases to be produced in women at menopause.

Apparently, women who produce higher than average amounts of androstenone are judged to be extremely attractive; they also have a strong libido. All things being equal, there may be a grain of truth in this claim. Indeed, it has been revealed that Brigitte Bardot radiates a musky aroma – not from a bottle of costly French perfume, but from her own enticing essence!

Most female pheromones, collectively called 'copulins', are so light and volatile that they can be diffused across a room. The relatively 'heavyweight' male pheromones (and the female secretions of androstenone) can only be transferred by intimate contact. This same pattern is seen in the insect and animal kingdoms – males pick up female aromas over vast distances, whereas females need to be 'caught' before they can respond to the male scent. Interestingly, butterflies often give off an aroma to attract a mate, and this luring scent may smell like roses, heliotrope and other flowers.

The quantity of pheromones produced by individuals can vary enormously. This may be the reason why an ordinary looking man or woman can sometimes possess an amazingly sexy aura, and why a perfect Adonis or Aphrodite may come over as somewhat bland. Indeed the writer Somerset Maugham, curious to know the secret of H. G. Wells's success with women reported, 'He was fat and homely. I once asked one of his mistresses what attracted her to him. I expected her to say his acute mind and sense of fun: not at all; she said that his body smelt of honey.'

More often, however, sexual chemistry between humans is less easy to explain. Pheromones apart, physical appearance is important (we tend to be especially attracted to those who resemble ourselves to a greater or lesser degree), as is personality, the tone of voice – and who knows what else besides. Such is the mystery of love!

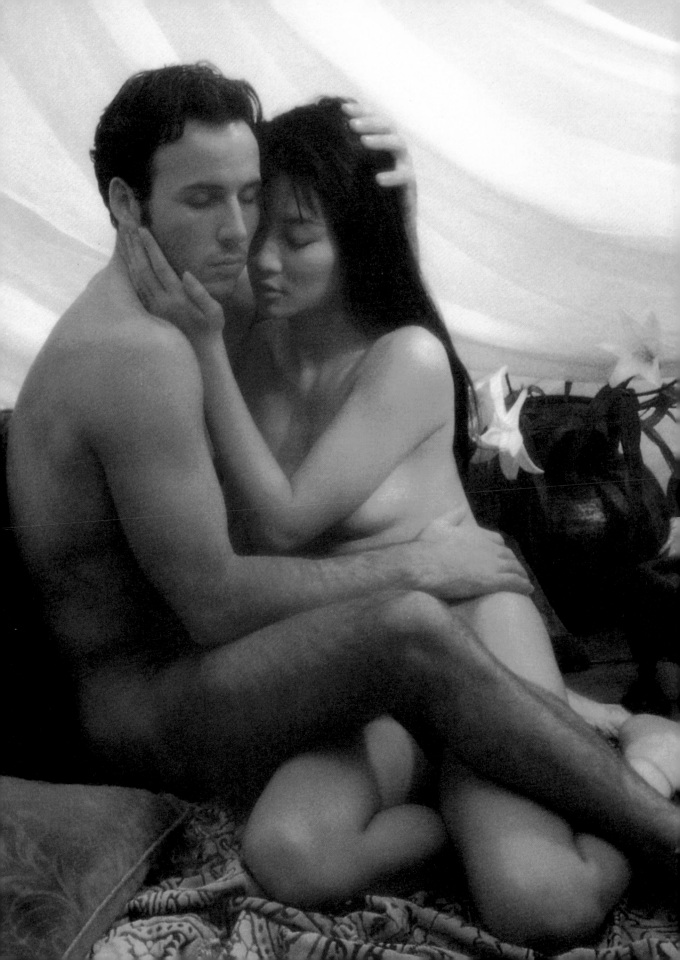

CHAPTER 2

Aromatherapy in Essence

What is understood by essence, in the pure sense as used by the medieval alchemists, for example, is the actual energy, the 'soul' of the plant.

Marguerite Maury

A Healing Art

People have always been intrigued by the seemingly magical properties of aromatic plants. As far back as any archaeologist can decipher, aromatic plants have been used, not only for culinary and medicinal purposes, but also for their ability to engender altered states of consciousness. It was found that burning some plant resins as incense made people feel relaxed or drowsy while other kinds of incense made them feel uplifted, even euphoric. The most precious of all gave rise to certain mystical states; these special aromatics were burned only by priests and priestesses during religious rites or for healing purposes. Since healing and religion were interrelated, the 'smoking' of sick people (often to exorcize evil spirits) became an important aspect of the healer's art.

The ancient Egyptians, however, are generally regarded as the true founders of aromatherapy as we know it. Apart from using aromatic oils for embalming and for religious ceremonies, the oils were employed for cosmetic and therapeutic purposes, with aromatic oil massage playing an important role. The Greeks and Romans were to follow suit, placing great emphasis on the aromatic bath, followed by massage, as a means of attaining good health, sexual vigour, and a sense of well-being.

Modern Aromatherapy

To cut a long aromatic history short, although the roots of this fascinating therapy lie buried in the depths of antiquity, the word 'aromatherapy' was first used in 1937 when the French cosmetic scientist René-Maurice Gattefossé wrote the first book on the subject. His interest was aroused when preliminary research revealed that the volatile extracts distilled from certain aromatic plants and trees had a profound effect on the skin. Although his initial research was confined to the cosmetic uses of essential oils, he soon realized that many had

powerful antiseptic and painkilling properties as well. The most remarkable instance of this was demonstrated to Gattefossé after his hand was severely burned in a laboratory explosion. He treated the wound with neat lavender essence, which immediately eased the pain. Moreover, the burn healed remarkably well, with no sign of infection, or even a scar to remind him of the accident.

Gattefossé also discovered that essential oils applied to the skin could be absorbed into the bloodstream, and then interact with the body's chemistry. The tiny aromatic molecules slip through the skin's hair follicles, which contain sebum, an oily liquid with which they have an affinity. From here they diffuse into the bloodstream or are taken up by the lymph and interstitial fluid (a liquid surrounding all body cells) to other parts of the body. If the skin is healthy, it takes about an hour for the oil to be absorbed; much longer if the skin is congested or if there is much subcutaneous fat. Traces of essential oil can often be detected in the urine an hour or two after application.

In fact, the ancients were well aware of the skin's ability to convey substances to the blood. The 'black witches' sometimes used poisonous ointments impregnated with extracts of hemlock, belladonna and other lethal plants, to see off their enemies.

Up until the early twentieth century, syphilis was treated by rubbing the body with mercury ointment. It was very difficult to judge the amount absorbed, which often resulted in some horrible side-effects. Even though the treatment killed many, it often succeeded in eradicating the infection in those with a stronger constitution. Administering drugs by inunction (through the skin) has been made safer recently with the introduction of measured doses. For example, oestrogen and trinitrin can be taken up through the skin in very gradual doses from a patch applied to the skin. Nicotine patches work under the same principle.

A great deal of interest in aromatherapy was kindled in France as a result of Gattefossé's work. Not only were the oils found to heal skin, they strengthened the body's immune defences. Moreover, Professor Paolo Rovesti of Milan, for example, demonstrated the psychotherapeutic effects of smelling essential oils. Using the essences produced from locally grown fruits such as bergamot, orange and lemon, he passed bits of cotton wool soaked in essential oil under the noses of his patients. The aromas, he said, helped to evoke and release suppressed memories and emotions that had detrimental effects on the psyche of these people.

The ex-army surgeon Dr Jean Valnet is credited with having contributed most to the medical assessment and acceptance of aromatherapy. Inspired by Gattefossé, he used essential oils to treat battle wounds of soldiers during the Second World War. Later, in his book, *Aromathérapie*, he describes how he successfully treated several long-term psychiatric patients with essential oils. These people also had physical symptoms caused by the side-effects of drugs they had been given to control their depression and hallucinations. They were gradually weaned off the drugs and treated both externally (aromatic baths and liniment rubs) and internally (by mouth or by interdermal injection) with essential oils. The treatment was reinforced with herbal remedies and a strict dietary regime. Both physical and mental symptoms were relieved, sometimes within days of discontinuing the drugs.

Due to the work of the early pioneers, several medical schools in France now include the study of essential oils as part of their curriculum. Moreover, a form of herbal medicine called phytotherapy, which features the use of essential oils, is also widely practised in France and many other countries in Europe.

In the 1950s, the Austrian-born biochemist Marguerite Maury introduced the idea of combining essential oils with massage. She was not happy with the idea of administering essential oils by mouth (as advocated by Valnet and others), but preferred to dilute them in vegetable oil and to massage them into the skin. Inspired by the methods used in traditional Tibetan medicine, she developed a special massage technique of applying the oils along the nerve centres of the spine. She also devised the 'individual prescription' – essences were chosen according to the individual physical and emotional needs of the recipient. Her clients, mainly wealthy women seeking rejuvenation, reported dramatic improvements in their skin condition as a result of her treatments. To their delight, there were also some interesting 'side-effects'; many experienced relief from rheumatic pain, heightened sexual pleasure, deeper sleep, and a generally improved mental state. The effects lasted weeks or sometimes months after treatments had finished.

More Than Skin Deep

Marguerite Maury opened an aromatherapy clinic in London in the early 1960s, thus spreading the word to Britain. Although her treatments were geared to 'beauty therapy' she knew that aromatherapy went much deeper. Indeed, she had discovered an important key to the art of true healing.

However, it could be argued that it was the British therapist Robert Tisserand who really put aromatherapy on the agenda. He is the author of *The Art of Aromatherapy*, one of the first books in English on the subject. He traces the history of healing with aromatic plants and discusses the therapeutic properties and applications of a number of essential oils. Although inspired by Marguerite Maury, it would be fair to say that this book above any other has sparked the greatest interest, world-wide, in the therapeutic properties of essential oils and aromatherapy in general.

The Nature of Essential Oils

Before we look more closely at the therapeutic actions of plant essences, we should discover what essential oils are and how they are captured. Essential oils are the odoriferous, volatile (evaporate readily) liquid components of aromatic plants, trees and grasses. They accumulate in specialized cells or in specific parts of the plant. They may be found in petals (rose), leaves (eucalyptus), wood (sandalwood), rind (lemon), seeds (caraway), roots (vetiver), rhizomes (ginger), resin (frankincense), and sometimes in more than one part of the plant. Lavender and peppermint, for example, both yield an essential oil from the flowers and leaves. The orange tree is particularly interesting, for it produces three different-smelling essences with differing properties from different parts of the plant – neroli (flowers), petitgrain (leaves) and orange (rind).

Although technically classified as oils, plant essences are quite different from ordinary 'fixed' oils such as sunflower or corn oil. Most have the consistency of water or alcohol. Others such as vetiver and myrrh are viscous, and rose otto is semi-solid at room temperature.

The quality of an essential oil depends on many interrelated factors: soil conditions, climate, altitude and the time of harvesting. Generally, the concentration of essential oil in plants is most abundant during warm weather and this is the best collecting time. However, the essential oil also moves around the plant according to both a daily and a seasonal cycle – individual plant species having their own idiosyncratic rhythm. The oil of jasmine, for instance, is most concentrated in the petals at night, which means the flowers must be picked before dawn. The oil of

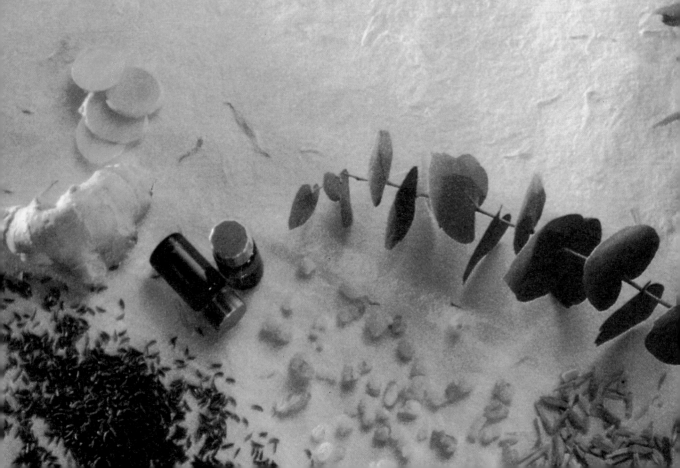

the damask rose, on the other hand, is most concentrated in the petals early in the morning.

Moreover, like wine, the quality and 'bouquet' of an essential oil will vary from year to year. Although some essences are very expensive, especially rose otto and neroli, they are highly concentrated substances; if used in the correct dilutions as advocated in Chapter 4, you will find that a little goes a long way.

Capturing Essential Oils

Most essential oils are captured by steam distillation, a process whose origins can be traced back to the Mesopotamians over five thousand years ago. Plant material is piled into a still and subjected to concentrated steam, which acts to release the essential oils from the plant cells. The aromatic vapour passes along a series of glass tubes which act as a condenser. The oil is then separated from the water by siphoning it off through a narrow-necked container. The remaining water may form beautifully fragrant by-products; rosewater, orange flower water and lavender water are well-known examples.

The oils of citrus fruits such as bergamot, lemon and lime are much easier to obtain. Indeed, the essence (the zest of the fruit) is found in such profusion that it sprays the surrounding air when the fruit is peeled. Citrus essences are captured by a simple process known as expression. Although this was once carried out by hand (by squeezing or pressing the rind), machines using centrifugal force are now used instead.

The most concentrated aromatic oils are produced by a complicated process known as volatile solvent extraction. This method is commonly used to obtain the fragrances of flowers such as jasmine, mimosa and carnation, whose exquisite fragrances are spoiled by the intense heat of steam distillation. Solvent extraction is the method favoured by the perfume industry. The resulting liquid is called an absolute. If solvent extraction is used with a resin (benzoin for example) the liquid is called a resinoid.

Strictly speaking, absolutes and resinoids are perfume materials rather than aromatherapy grade essential oils. Unfortunately, they often contain traces of the chemical solvent (hexane or petroleum ether, for example) used in the extraction process, and this can cause skin irritation in a few people. Although I no longer use absolutes or resinoids in professional aromatherapy treatments, there may be a place for their use in perfume-making or in room scents – as reflected in the practical sections of this book. However, there is a choice of aromatic materials, which means you can avoid the use of solvent extracted oils and the risk of skin irritations should you so wish.

Natural Versus Synthetic

Although chemists have tried to duplicate essential oils in the laboratory, synthetic or 'nature identical' oils are not the same as pure, natural essential oils. Any synthetic will carry with it a small percentage of undesirable substances which are not found in the essential oil.

Moreover, a synthetic oil lacks the vital enzymes and probably a multitude of other substances as yet undiscovered, which are found in plants. Indeed, 'nature identical' aromatics never smell exactly the same as the real thing. Something is always missing. Synthetic aromatics are also more likely to cause skin and respiratory irritation.

Above all, however, the use of laboratory chemicals runs counter to the philosophy of aromatherapy whose aim is to use only organic essences – that is to say, essential oils born of the synergy of earth, air, sunlight and rain, rather than the synthesis of white coats and test tubes – and here we must leave the argument! Make sure that the essential oils you buy are pure undiluted essential oils (*see the Appendix for a list of stockists*).

Essential Oils in Action

A plant produces essential oils for its own survival: to influence growth and reproduction; to attract pollinating insects; to repel predators; and to protect itself from disease – they can do as much for people too. Studies have shown that the essential oils of lavender and neroli, for example, are cytophylactic: they stimulate the growth of healthy skin cells. Moreover, a great many essential oils, when applied to the skin (suitably diluted in vegetable carrier oil) encourage the elimination of cellular wastes and support the function of blood capillaries. In other words, they improve the circulation thus imparting a naturally acquired healthy glow.

According to Dr Jean Valnet, the essential oils of rose, chamomile and cypress influence hormonal secretions, thus exerting a beneficial effect on the reproductive system. A few essences have been credited with the ability to improve the quality and flow of mothers' milk – fennel, caraway and anise, for example. Indeed, for centuries herbalists have used the seeds of these plants for that purpose. If for some reason the milk needs to be stopped, the essential oils of sage, peppermint and parsley will have the opposite effect and will help to diminish the flow of milk.

Many oils, notably rosemary, eucalyptus and geranium, will kill head lice (the human equivalent to an attack of greenfly). While all oils are antiseptic to a greater or lesser degree, some have antiviral properties as well – the essential oils of tea tree, clove, camphor, lavender and eucalyptus are good examples.

As for 'attracting pollinating insects', for centuries aromatic plant extracts have been used for their erogenous effects. Indeed, no love philtre was deemed potent without them. Some of the most renowned aphrodisiacs include rose, sandalwood, jasmine and ylang ylang.

Unlike a chemical drug, which may contain a single active principle, an essential oil may be composed of hundreds of chemical components such as terpenes, esters, ketones, phenols, aldehydes and oxides. This explains why a single essential oil can effect numerous different changes. Whether absorbed through the skin or inhaled (aromatic molecules can also reach the bloodstream via the lungs), once in the bloodstream and body fluids, the aromatic molecules exert their therapeutic effect – even though the amount absorbed may be very tiny indeed. However, the efficacy of the oils may be due to the fact that aromatherapy treatments are given once or twice a week over a period of not less than one month. In the manner of a biocatalyst, the oils gently stimulate the body's own self-healing ability. Having triggered the desired effect, they are then rapidly excreted – without having changed in themselves.

Another curious property of plant essences is

that although specific essences, say melissa or neroli, are known to alleviate emotional shock, or others, say peppermint or ginger, are good stimulants for lethargic states, unlike pharmaceutical drugs, some also appear to have more than one action on the nervous system. So a person suffering from exhaustion as a result of hyperanxiety can be both calmed and stimulated by sniffing peppermint. Similarly, researchers in eastern Europe have found that garlic oil (taken orally in capsule form) has the ability to raise abnormally low blood pressure and to lower blood pressure that is too high.

Just how essential oils (and also many herbal remedies) exert such a 'normalizing' effect remains a mystery, though most aromatherapists believe it is the result of a special synergy that only nature can orchestrate. The effect is of the whole essence being greater than the sum of its equal parts. In other words, the naturally occurring interaction of biochemicals is far more efficacious than the chemist might expect of the essence – taking into account the combined chemical constituents of the oil.

Essential Oils and Vaginal Secretions

An interesting 'side-effect' of using essential oils in general (in baths and body massage applications) has been reported by British aromatherapist Valerie Ann Worwood: she says they increase the amount of vaginal secretions. Although this has not been borne out by my own experience, given that many essences influence hormonal activity, it is possible that they may also influence vaginal secretion. Those who may benefit most are women troubled by vaginal dryness during menopause – a common symptom thought to be caused by the drastic reduction in oestrogen levels at this time. Although vaginal dryness in healthy younger women is sometimes caused by taking the Pill, the amount of secretion during love-making is largely dependent on the degree of sexual excitement.

Although the evidence is circumstantial, the essences V. A. Worwood credits with being especially helpful for vaginal dryness include: geranium, sandalwood, rose otto, clary sage, ylang ylang, lavender, neroli and cypress. What is certain, however, is that essential oils rubbed into the skin subtly perfume vaginal secretions, and other body fluids such as sweat and urine within a few hours of use.

The Mind and Emotions

No matter what you may have heard to the contrary, the emotional effect of different essential oils is highly subjective. The images and feelings an aroma may evoke (or dispel) cannot be predicted. Yet still we hear that rose will magic away jealousy, chamomile will sweeten dreams, and cedarwood will dampen down anger. The truth is that any oil can bring about any desired emotional change if we truly believe it has the power to do so; the role played by the power of suggestion should never be underestimated in the art of healing. An aroma is a self-healing tool which can be used to focus the attention on a specific area of negativity – and this is the first step towards letting it go of a negative emotion.

Idiosyncratic responses apart, most aromas (including synthetic scents) exert a generalized effect on the central nervous system, albeit a very subtle influence. Some may bring about a state of relaxation, others may make us feel more alert. Indeed, the mental and physical effects of odour can be measured by EEG (electroencephalograph) scanning equipment. Interestingly, olfactory experiments carried out at Warwick University (England) revealed that if we dislike an aroma intensely enough we can block its effect on the central nervous system.

So for an aroma to be of any benefit it must at least be perceived as acceptable. This being the case, studies have shown that sandalwood, chamomile and vetiver, for example, are mildly sedative – they produce alpha, theta and delta brainwave patterns. Other aromas such as black pepper, rosemary and coriander produce beta brainwaves indicating a state of alertness. A few oils have been credited with exerting a 'normalizing' effect – they can gently stimulate people who feel lethargic, and lower anxiety levels in those who feel tense and nervy – bergamot and lavender are especially helpful.

A Pleasurable Therapy

Aromatherapy, as it is practised in most countries, is primarily a hands-on therapy. It combines the physical and emotional effects of gentle massage with the medicinal and psychotherapeutic properties of plant essences. It also involves several other methods of application – including baths, mood-enhancing room scents, and the use of aromatic lotions and potions. Aromatherapy is also practised without the use of massage in France, where the main application is oral dosage. In this instance, it could be said that the word 'aromatherapy' is something of a misnomer, since the oils are chosen for their pharmacological properties rather than the subtle effect of the aroma on the mind.

Clearly, as far as aromatherapy is concerned, there is no truth in the age-old belief that a certain amount of discomfort must be felt if it is to do us any good. Indeed, the more wonderful the experience, the more healing the effect. This view was shared by the ancient Greek physician Asclepiades, who advocated the use of massage, aromatic baths, music and perfume to soothe away the stresses and strains of life – even wine had a place in his Elysian regime! It is easy to understand how aromatherapy can be adopted by couples wishing to use massage combined with essential oils to foster a more sensuous emotional and sexual relationship.

The Individual Prescription

Aromatherapy is both a preventive therapy and a healing tool in its own right. Its main aim is to strengthen the body's immune defences. When applied with skilled, sensitive touch, aromatherapy is one of the finest treatments available to help soothe away the detrimental effects of stress. Stress, as we know, has a damaging effect on general health as well as having a detrimental effect on the libido – the last thing an overstressed partner wants is sex. Stress relief, therefore, is perhaps the first step in restoring an interest in love-making; what better treatment than a soothing and restoring aromatherapy massage given by a loving partner.

Indeed, aromatherapy is a marvellous adjunct to most treatments – from the nurturing of a loving sexual relationship to medical herbalism, acupuncture, or even orthodox medicine. The tender loving care approach to treatment is gaining medical acceptance.

Of course, it is important for both aromatherapist and client to feel at ease with one another – especially when massage is involved – for the treatment to be entirely successful. This is as true for two loving partners as it is between any caring professional and client. To get the most out of any treatment, trust, warmth and confidence must be present. If this sounds unlikely, consider whether you would choose to go more than once to a dentist or a doctor whose manner and touch made you feel uncomfortable. In fact, any health practitioner who can make you feel at ease by radiating genuine warmth is going to make you feel better even before the treatment is given.

There are some aromatherapists, however, who go out of their way to play down the relaxation aspect of aromatherapy in order to make it appear more 'scientific', thus underestimating the self-healing power of relaxation. They will use computerized cross-referenced charts to ascertain the 'right' oil for the individual and their physical ailment (as if the two were separate). In doing so, it is often forgotten that individuals respond very differently to the same essential oils, both physically and emotionally. As French aromatherapy doctors have discovered through clinical tests what works for one person does not necessarily work for another – something a computer cannot work out.

It is particularly important, therefore that both you and your partner like the fragrance of any combinations of essential oils that you might use in either sensual or relaxing aromatherapy massage. For this we may conclude that the intuitive approach to aromatherapy, which involves 'a meeting of two minds' based on knowledge, feelings and aroma preferences is (whether between two loving partners, or between aromatherapist and client) at least as accurate (or as hit-or-miss) as the cross reference, computerized, high-tech approach to choosing oils.

An Holistic Approach

According to the philosophy of holistic or whole person healing, almost every malady known to humanity is the result of emotional disharmony at some level. When we are distressed we become more susceptible to illness – we also become more accident-prone at such times. Indeed, the visionary physician Dr Edward Bach (founder of the Bach Flower Remedy system of healing in the 1930s) was also aware of the interrelatedness of body and mind. He maintained that 'disease is a consolidation of a mental state'. Although this view was virtually unheard of in orthodox medicine, Hippocrates, the father of medicine, and many other ancient physicians of renown in both the Western and Eastern healing traditions, had reached the same understanding. Nowadays this concept is grounded in the new science known as psychoneuroimmunology.

Any therapy which enables a person to relax deeply, to let go of all their cares – even for just a while – is potentially powerful enough to activate self-healing processes. Moreover, true healing is about learning to give and receive unconditional love – that which transcends romantic love – the ultimate healing force.

Unfortunately it is beyond the scope of this book to go deeply into the philosophy of holism. But suffice to say here, although some people are born healthier than others, most of us can become healthier and prevent the onset of many physical and emotional disorders such as stress-related sexual difficulties, heart disease, maturity onset diabetes, and the many other 'diseases of civilization'. The key to good health and a sense of well-being lies in the realization that we need not become helpless victims of our own distress. There are many ways in which we can approach improving our own physical and emotional well-being.

To a large extent, of course, our health is dependent on the quality of the food we eat, the water we drink and the air we breathe. Perhaps even more importantly, we need to nurture the spiritual aspect of 'self', for we are more than a body and a mind. The spiritual aspect is hard to define, but is tied up with our relationship with ourselves, our partners and other significant people in our lives. It also involves our sense of having a purpose and meaning, of having a place in the world. Without purpose we become depressed or apathetic; life then appears bleak and meaningless. So true healing can only come about if we address the interrelated aspects of our being as a whole: the body, mind and spirit. Although the mind/spirit aspect has the ultimate directive, whatever affects one aspect – the body, the mind or the spirit – affects the whole.

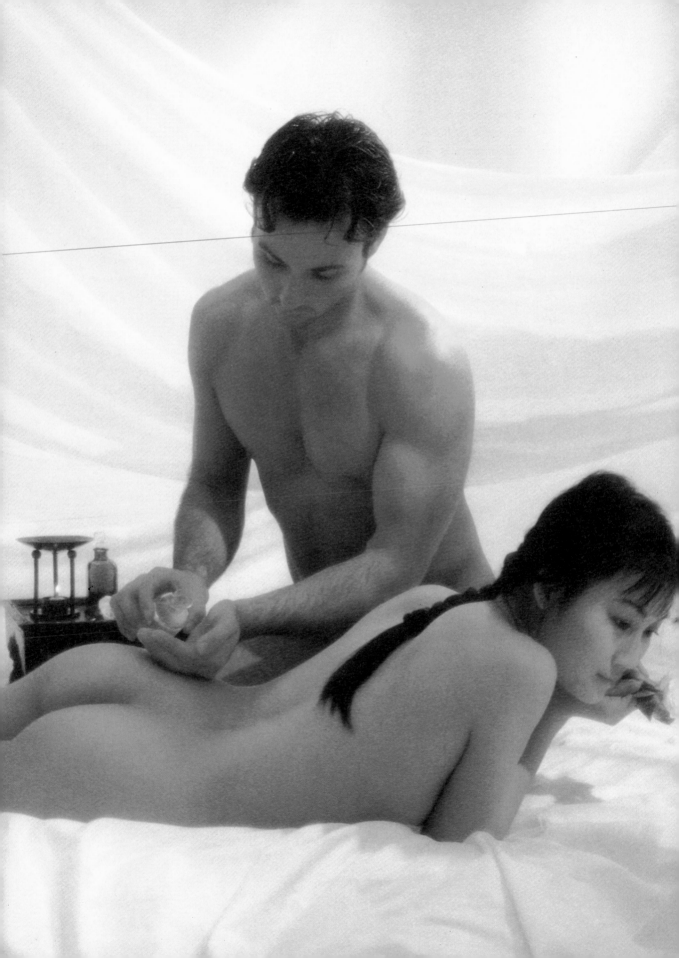

CHAPTER 3

Aphrodite's Pharmacy

Aphrodite went away to Cyprus, and entered her fragrant temple at Paphos, where she had a precinct and a fragrant altar. After going inside she closed the bright doors, and the Graces gave her a bath, they oiled her with sacred olive-oil, the kind that the gods always have on, that pleasant ambrosia that she was perfumed with.

The Homeric Hymns

Exploring Aphrodite's Pharmacy

The aromatics featured here are the most popular oils used in aromatherapy and natural perfumery. However, on first acquaintance, some may smell rather strange – natural aromatics are very different from the synthetic fragrances to which many people have become accustomed. The main reason for the 'strangeness' of essential oils is that they are highly concentrated substances. It is only when they are suitably diluted that they begin to resemble the characteristic aromas of the plants from which they are obtained. But even then, a captured essence will never smell exactly the same as that radiated by the living plant. Unfortunately, no matter how sophisticated the extraction process, the fragrance shape shifts to a greater or lesser degree. In fact, as soon as the plant material is collected, the aroma will change.

Yet just as we can learn to appreciate good wine or unusual foods, we can become enamoured of the beauty of natural fragrances. Indeed, once weaned on to naturals, synthetic fragrances may even seem like an unpleasant nostril-stinging assault.

Individual Profiles

Let us begin to reveal the contents of Aphrodite's pharmacy. Each profile begins with a brief outline of the origin of the plant and its essential oil, followed by a description of the oil itself. Most essences have the consistency of water or alcohol; a few could be described as viscous. Following the outline of the plant is a description of the odour itself and its effect. Although we cannot be certain of the emotional effect of an aroma on the individual, the most common responses are listed.

Also included is a list of the main therapeutic properties of each oil. However, do remember that sensual aromatherapy is much more about choosing mood-enhancing aromas according to your intuitive responses, your aroma preferences, rather than the pharmacological properties of the plant essences. Should you wish to use the oils for a specific problem, do seek the advice of a qualified aromatherapist and/or obtain an informative book on the subject (*see the suggested reading list in the Appendix*).

The blending hints will be helpful when you come to experiment with your own fragrant compositions. Although there are no hard and fast rules (almost any oil will blend with another if skillfully mixed in the correct proportions), the information is included just to point you in the right direction. The myth and magic section can be taken as an interesting aside, while the price, availability and cautions sections are self-explanatory.

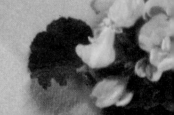

Enchanting Florals

These aromatic oils have been captured principally from flowers, and their fragrances are those of their blooms. The most obvious and perhaps most enchanting of these oils comes from the rose — the flower of love.

Rose Otto
Rosa damascena

Source: Distillation of the fresh petals of the damask rose, which is native to the Orient, but is now cultivated mainly in Bulgaria. Rosewater is produced as a by-product of the distillation process.

Nature: An almost colourless liquid which becomes semi-solid in coolish temperatures. To make the essence liquid, rub the bottle between the palms of your hands, or place in a cup of lukewarm water for about half a minute. Never place the bottle in very hot water as the heat will eventually cause the oil to deteriorate.

Odour description and effect: A sweet, mellow aroma with a hint of vanilla and clove. It engenders a warm, heady sensation. The aroma also has antidepressant properties and is a reputed aphrodisiac.

Therapeutic uses: Skin care (most skin types), thread veins, eczema, palpitations, hay fever, poor circulation, irregular menstruation, uterine disorders, depression and other stress-related disorders.

Blends well with: Most oils, especially citrus essences and sandalwood. Use in tiny amounts as the oil has a high odour intensity.

Myth and magic: The word rosa derives from the Greek *rodon* (red), and the rose of the ancients was a deep crimson, which gave rise to the myth of its springing from the blood of Adonis. Sacred to Aphrodite, no love philtre nor alluring perfume was deemed potent without a few precious drops of the essence – or at least a sprinkling of rosewater. Sappho, the ancient Greek poetess, crowned the rose 'Queen of all flowers'.

Price and availability: Very costly; rose otto is usually only available from specialist mail order suppliers.

CAUTIONS: Avoid use during early pregnancy.

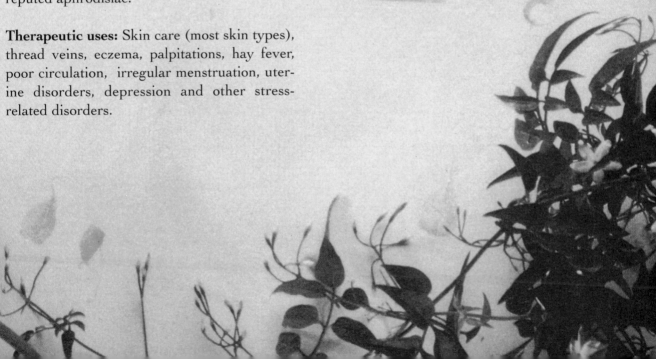

Rose Absolute
Rosa centifolia

Source: Solvent extraction of the fresh petals of the flower native to the Middle East, but now cultivated mainly in Morocco and France from hybrid roses. This oil is labelled 'absolute' and should not be confused with rose otto – the only rose oil captured by steam distillation.

Nature: A yellowy-orange, viscous liquid.

Odour description and effect: A sweet, mellow, spicy-floral fragrance similar to rose otto, though much lighter. It has a calming, yet uplifting effect; a reputed aphrodisiac.

Therapeutic uses: As for rose otto.

Blends well with: Most oils, especially citrus essences and sandalwood.

Myth and magic: As for rose otto.

Price and availability: Very costly. More easily obtained from mail order sources.

CAUTIONS: Avoid use during pregnancy.

Jasmine
Jasminum officinale

Source: Solvent extraction of the night-scented flowers of the evergreen climber native to China, India and western Asia. Most of the oil is produced in Egypt and France.

Nature: The absolute is amber and viscous.

Odour description and effect: A warm, floral scent with a musky undertone. The tenacious aroma is warming, stimulating and an anti-depressant; a reputed aphrodisiac.

Therapeutic uses: Depression, nervous exhaustion and stress-related conditions.

Blends well with: Other florals, citrus essences, clary sage, sandalwood.

Myth and magic: The flower is sacred to Kama, the Hindu god of love.

Price and availability: Very costly, most easily obtained from specialist mail order suppliers.

CAUTIONS: May irritate sensitive skin.

Geranium
Pelargonium graveolens

Source: Distillation of the leaves, stalks and flowers of a shrub native to South Africa. Most of the oil is produced in Réunion and Egypt.

Nature: A greenish watery liquid.

Odour description and effect: A piercingly sweet rose-like scent with a hint of mint. Its odour effect is refreshing and uplifting.

Therapeutic uses: Skin care (congested skin conditions), dermatitis, eczema, burns, head lice, ringworm, wounds, cellulite, poor circulation, premenstrual and menopausal symptoms, nervous tension and stress-related conditions.

Blends well with: Bergamot and other citrus oils, lavender, clary sage, clove, patchouli, vetiver, sandalwood, jasmine, juniper, neroli.

Myth and magic: Modern magicians use the oil in rituals invoking love and happiness.

Price and availability: Medium price range.

CAUTIONS: May irritate very sensitive skin.

Neroli (Orange Blossom)
Citrus aurantium

Source: Distillation of the blossom of the bitter orange tree which is native to the Far East, but cultivated for its oil in the Mediterranean, Morocco and Egypt. A solvent extraction is available and is known as orange flower absolute. Orange flower water is produced as a by-product of the distillation process.

Nature: A pale yellow liquid with the consistency of water or alcohol. The absolute is a dark amber viscous liquid.

Odour description and effect: A sweet floral fragrance with a bitter undertone. The aroma of the absolute is much closer to that of the fresh orange blossom, warm and sweetly floral. The odour effect of both neroli and orange flower absolute is uplifting and calming; an antidepressant and a reputed aphrodisiac.

Therapeutic uses: Skin care, stretch marks, palpitations, poor circulation, diarrhoea, anxiety, depression, premenstrual syndrome, shock and stress-related disorders. The absolute is best used as a perfume or room scent for healing distressing emotions.

Blends well with: Citrus essences, chamomile, clary sage, jasmine, geranium, coriander, lavender, rose, ylang ylang.

Myth and magic: Said to take its name from the Roman emperor Nero, though others argue that it is named for a sixteenth-century prince of Nerola, Flavio Orsini, whose wife perfumed her bath and gloves with the essence.

Price and availability: Very costly. May be available from health shops diluted in a base oil. The absolute is easier to obtain from specialist mail order suppliers.

Ylang Ylang
Cananga odorata

Source: Distillation of the flowers of the tall tropical tree native to Asia. Most of the oil is produced in Madagascar, Réunion and Comoro Islands. There are four grades of ylang ylang which should be labelled: ylang ylang extra, then ylang ylang one, two and three. Always use the more expensive ylang ylang extra, which has a vastly superior aroma. This is because it is collected from the 'first running' of the distillation process; the plant material is distilled two or three more times to obtain the lower grades.

Nature: A pale yellow liquid with the consistency of water or alcohol.

Odour description and effect: An intensely sweet, floral scent reminiscent of almonds and jasmine combined. A heady, antidepressant aroma; a reputed aphrodisiac.

Therapeutic uses: Promotes healthy hair growth, high blood pressure, palpitations, depression, insomnia, nervous tension and stress-related disorders.

Blends well with: Other florals, citrus essences, vetiver, frankincense, geranium.

Myth and magic: Name means 'flower of flowers'. In Indonesia the blooms are scattered over the beds of newly married couples on their wedding night to promote sexual desire and to ensure that the marriage will be blessed with many children. As well as being regarded as an aphrodisiac, the fragrance is said to bring about a state of peacefulness.

Price and availability: Medium price range. Lower grades widely available. The best grade is available from mail order suppliers.

Eleusinian Woods

*The following oils have been distilled from the
roots, leaves and woods of evergreen trees. Their fragrance, as a result,
is that of a cool, refreshing forest.*

Pine, Scots
Pinus sylvestris

Source: Distillation of the needles of the evergreen tree native to Scotland and Norway. Most of the oil is produced in the eastern USA from cultivated trees.

Nature: A colourless to pale yellow liquid with the consistency of water or alcohol.

Odour description and effect: A dry, balsamic, turpentine-like aroma. Its odour effect is cooling, comforting and refreshing.

Therapeutic uses: Excessive perspiration, arthritis, muscular aches and pains, poor circulation, rheumatism, respiratory ailments, cystitis, colds and flu, fatigue, nervous exhaustion.

Blends well with: Bergamot, lemon, cedarwood juniper, rosemary, lavender.

Myth and magic: The Greek god of wine, Dionysus, is also associated with the pine tree. Paintings often depict the god holding a wand tipped with a pine cone.

Price and availability: Medium price range; widely available.

CAUTIONS: Use in low concentrations as it may irritate sensitive skin.

Cedarwood, Atlas
Cedrus atlantica

Source: Distillation of the wood, stumps and sawdust from the evergreen tree native to the Atlas Mountains of Algeria. Most of the oil is produced in Morocco.

Nature: A dark amber liquid with the consistency of water or alcohol.

Odour description and effect: A camphoraceous tinge with a sweet-woody undertone. Aroma improves as it ages. Its effect is calming and antidepressant; a reputed aphrodisiac.

Therapeutic uses: Skin care (oily skin and acne), dandruff, eczema, oily skin, psoriasis, arthritis, rheumatism, respiratory disorders, cystitis, premenstrual distress, loss of menstruation outside pregnancy, nervous tension and stress-related disorders.

Blends well with: Bergamot, clary sage, cypress, juniper, frankincense, neroli, rose, jasmine, rosemary, vetiver, ylang ylang.

Myth and magic: Believed to be the first oil to be distilled in primitive clay pots by the ancient Egyptians. Used for embalming, medicinal purposes, skin care, perfumery and as a sacred incense material.

Price and availability: Lowest price range; widely available.

CAUTIONS: Not to be used during pregnancy.

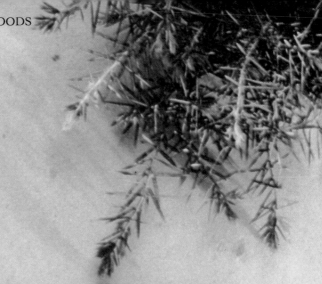

Cypress
Cupressus sempervirens

Source: Distillation of the needles, twigs and cones of the tall conifer tree native to the eastern Mediterranean. Most of the oil is produced in France, Spain and Morocco.

Nature: A pale yellow liquid with the consistency of water or alcohol.

Odour description and effect: A woody-balsamic aroma, its effect is cooling and calming. Aroma can engender a peaceful, spacious sensation in those who feel pressurized.

Therapeutic uses: Skin care (oily skin), acne, haemorrhoids, excessive perspiration, gum disorders, varicose veins, wounds, respiratory disorders, circulatory problems, fluid retention, cellulite, rheumatic complaints, excessive menstruation, menopausal problems, nervous tension and stress.

Blends well with: Bergamot and the other citrus oils, clary sage, pine, juniper, lavender, sandalwood.

Myth and magic: A popular oil in ancient Egypt; papyri record its medicinal uses. The tree is sacred to the Roman god Pluto, ruler of the underworld, thus the frequency of the tree in cemeteries. For magical purposes, the somewhat solemn aroma is said to engender inner strength and quietude and is particularly helpful during periods of transition such as the parting of friends, the loss of a loved one, or the ending of a relationship.

Price and availability: Medium price range; widely available.

Petitgrain
Citrus aurantium

Source: Distillation of the leaves and twigs of the bitter orange tree native to southern China and north-east India. Most of the oil is produced in France.

Nature: A pale yellow liquid with the consistency of water or alcohol.

Odour description and effect: A fresh, woody, bitter-sweet aroma like neroli, but less refined. Its odour effect is refreshing and uplifting.

Therapeutic uses: Skin care (oily skin), nervous exhaustion and stress-related disorders.

Blends well with: Lavender, rosemary, bergamot, neroli, clary sage, jasmine, clove and geranium.

Myth and magic: Not known to the ancients. Is a classic eau-de-cologne ingredient.

Price and availability: Lowest price range; widely available.

Sandalwood
Santalum album

Source: Distillation of the roots and heartwood of the small evergreen tree native to tropical Asia. The best quality oil comes from Mysore in India. Not to be confused with West Indian Sandalwood or Amyris oil (*Amyris balsamifera*). Though less expensive, it has a different odour of poor tenacity.

Nature: A pale yellow, slightly viscous oil.

Odour description and effect: A warm, soft sweet-woody scent of excellent tenacity. The fragrance becomes more mellow as the oil ages. The odour effect is calming, sensual and anti-depressant; often regarded as the most potent aphrodisiac of the plant kingdom.

Therapeutic uses: Skin care (for excessively oily and excessively dry skin), respiratory ailments, nausea, cystitis, depression, insomnia, stress-related disorders.

Blends well with: Rose, clove, lavender, bergamot, vetiver, patchouli, jasmine, black pepper.

Myth and magic: One of the most ancient perfumes. Women in Burma, on the last day of the year, sprinkle people in the street with a mixture of rosewater and sandalwood essence to wash away the sins of the year. In magic, the oil is said to predispose the mind and body to the experience of sexual ecstasy.

Price and availability: High price range. Available from health shops and other retailers.

Enigmatic Resins

These oils are derived from the resins and gums of various trees and exotic plants. Their fragrances are dark and mysterious, ancient and unforgettable.

Vanilla
Vanilla planifolia

Source: Solvent extraction of the vanillin crystals which form on fermented vanilla beans. The plant is an herbaceous climbing orchid native to Mexico. It is cultivated mainly in Madagascar, Tahiti, Mexico and on the Comoro Islands.

Nature: A viscous dark-brown liquid.

Odour description and effect: A rich, sweet, balsamic aroma. The odour effect is warming, comforting and uplifting. It is also thought to be an aphrodisiac.

Therapeutic uses: Not generally used in aromatherapy. Use it as a room scent.

Blends well with: Rose, neroli, frankincense, sandalwood, vetiver, clove, ylang ylang, lime.

Myth and magic: In magic, vanilla is an ingredient in love philtres.

Price and availability: Very costly. The resinoid is extremely hard to obtain and very costly when available. The vanilla formulas suggested in this book contain the home-made infused oil or a water extraction of the pods. The oil is only available from a very few mail order suppliers.

Elemi
Canaraium luzonicum

Source: Distillation of the gum exuded from this tall tree native to the Philippines and the Moluccas.

Nature: A pale yellow colourless liquid with the consistency of water or alcohol.

Odour description and effect: A tenacious, spicy-balsamic aroma with a geranium-like overtone. The odour effect is both stimulating and warming.

Therapeutic uses: Rheumatic conditions, respiratory disorders, skin infections and nervous exhaustion.

Blends well with: Citrus essences, frankincense, rosemary, lavender, cinnamon, clove, coriander, geranium. Use in the lowest concentration as the oil has a high odour intensity.

Myth and magic: One of the aromatics used by the ancient Egyptians for embalming purposes. Its name in Arabic means 'as above, so below', which indicates its use in magical rituals for bringing about spiritual balance. The oil is also an excellent meditation aid, engendering clarity of thought combined with a sense of calm.

Price and availability: Medium price range; not very widely available. More easily obtainable from specialist mail order suppliers.

Frankincense
Boswellia carteri, B. thurifera

Source: Distillation of the gum exuded from the small tree native to north-east Africa.

Nature: A colourless to pale yellow liquid with the consistency of water or alcohol.

Odour description and effect: A warm, balsamic fragrance with a hint of lemon and camphor. The aroma improves greatly as the oil ages. The odour effect is warming, head clearing and calming. A popular oil for use during meditation.

Therapeutic uses: Skin care (particularly ageing skin), acne, abscesses, scars, wounds, haemorrhoids, respiratory ailments, nervous tension and stress-related disorders.

Blends well with: Citrus oil, spice oils, basil, lavender, neroli, rose, sandalwood and vetiver.

Myth and magic: This oil is also known as olibanum. Frankincense, along with sandalwood, cedarwood and myrrh, was highly prized by the ancients. It was the substance most frequently burned as holy incense. In magic, the vaporized oil is said to predispose mind and body to sexual ecstasy.

Price and availability: High price range. May be available from health shops and other retailers. Obtainable from mail order suppliers.

Potent Herbs

*Herbs have been used for medicinal and culinary purposes
for thousands of years. Their use as the source of therapeutic
essential oils may well be as ancient.*

Lavender
Lavandula angustifolia

Source: Distillation of the fresh flowering tops of the shrub native to the Mediterranean. The plant is cultivated all over the world, although most of the oil is produced in France, Spain and Bulgaria.

Nature: A colourless to pale yellow liquid with the consistency of water or alcohol.

Odour description and effect: A sweet, floral-herbaceous aroma. The odour effect is uplifting, calming and refreshing. Although not generally regarded as an aphrodisiac, occasionally you may come across a batch of lavender oil with a sensual honey-like undertone. Unfortunately, this is the luck of the draw since it is impossible to predict what an individual harvest may produce.

Therapeutic uses: Skin care (all skin types), acne, athlete's foot, burns, dandruff, earache, inflammations, insect bites and stings, insect repellent, head lice, psoriasis, ringworm, scabies, sunburn, wounds, respiratory ailments, cystitis, premenstrual syndrome, colds and flu, depression, headache and other stress-related conditions.

Blends well with: Most oils, especially citrus and floral.

Myth and magic: The name comes from the Latin *lavare*, which means 'to wash'. This is because the Romans used to steep the leaves and stems of the plant in their bath water and thus began the association of lavender with freshness that has lasted to this day. In North Africa, women use the plant as an amulet against maltreatment from their husbands. For magical purposes, lavender is used for invoking good health, tranquillity and psychic protection.

Price and availability: Lowest price range; widely available.

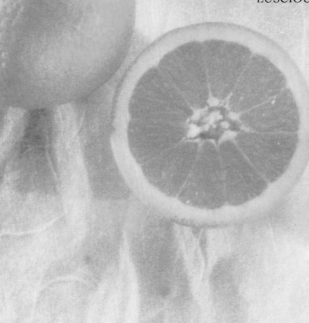

Myth and magic: The name *liminum* is derived from the Arabic *limun* or *lilnu*, which in turn probably comes from the Sanskrit *nimbuka*. Lemons were rare in ancient Greece and Rome, but the peel was used to perfume clothes and as a pesticide. It was not until the fourth century that the Romans began cultivating lemons on a large scale. The trees were also planted in the Sahara by Arab invaders in the eighth and ninth centuries. For magical purposes, the essence can be vaporized for self-purification and to inspire happiness.

Price and availability: Lowest price range; widely available.

CAUTIONS: Do not apply to the skin shortly before exposure to sunlight as it may cause brown blotching. Use in the lowest concentration as it may irritate the skin. This oil has a short shelf-life, so buy in small quantities and use within six to nine months.

Lemon
Citrus limon

Source: Expression of the outer part of the fresh peel of the fruit from the small evergreen tree native to Asia. Most of the oil is produced in the Mediterranean countries, especially Spain and Portugal.

Nature: A pale yellow liquid with the consistency of water or alcohol.

Odour description and effect: A sharp, fresh citrus scent. Its odour effect is refreshing, uplifting and antidepressant, like the fresh fruit.

Therapeutic uses: Skin care (oily skin conditions), arthritis, cellulite, high blood pressure, poor circulation, rheumatism, respiratory disorders, colds and flu, depression.

Blends well with: Other citrus essences, all florals, frankincense, juniper.

Orange, Sweet
Citrus aurantium

Source: Expression of the fresh ripe peel of the fruit from the small evergreen tree native to the Far East. Most of the oil is produced in Italy, Tunisia, Morocco and France. An inferior oil is distilled from the fruit pulp, so always ask for the more expensive expressed oil.

Nature: A pale yellow liquid with the consistency of water or alcohol.

Odour description and effect: A sweet, warm citrus scent. The aroma is uplifting and cheery.

Therapeutic uses: Palpitations, colds and flu, fluid retention, nervous exhaustion and depression.

Blends well with: Other citrus oils, floral essences, spice oils, clary sage, lavender and frankincense.

Myth and magic: The name is derived from the Sanskrit *nagaranga* through the Arabic *naranji*. The first mention of the fruit appears in the writings of the Arabs; the time and method of its first cultivation in Europe is unknown. For magical purposes, orange, in common with other citrus essences, is said to dispel depression and to engender happiness. The cheerful aroma of orange has the added charm of inspiring frivolity.

Price and availability: Lowest price range; widely available.

CAUTIONS: Do not apply to the skin shortly before exposure to sunlight as it may cause brown blotching. Use in the lowest concentration as it may irritate the skin. The oil has a short shelf-life, so buy in small quantities and use within six to nine months.

Mandarin
Citrus reticulata, C. nobilis

Source: Expression of the peel of the fruit from the small evergreen tree native to southern China and the Far East. Most of the oil is produced in Italy, Cyprus and Greece.

Nature: A yellow-orange liquid with the consistency of water or alcohol.

Odour description and effect: An intensely sweet citrus aroma. Its odour effect is soothing, uplifting and cheery.

Therapeutic uses: Stretch marks, cellulite, digestive problems, fluid retention, insomnia, nervous tension.

Blends well with: Other citrus essences, spice oils, neroli, ylang ylang, frankincense.

Myth and magic: The name is thought to have derived from the fact that the fruits were a traditional gift to the mandarins of China. Others are of the opinion that the shape of the fruit recalled the buttons on the hats of those imperial dignitaries. The fruit was brought to Europe in 1805 and to America some forty years later, where it was renamed the tangerine. For magical purposes, the essence of mandarin, like orange, is said to inspire feelings of happiness and frivolity.

Price and availability: Lowest price range. Often available from health shops and other retail outlets.

CAUTIONS: Do not apply to the skin shortly before exposure to sunlight as it may cause brown blotching. Use in the lowest concentrations as it may irritate the skin. The oil has a short shelf-life, so buy in small quantities and use within six to nine months.

Bergamot
Citrus bergamia

Source: Obtained by expression of the rind of the small orange-like fruit native to Italy.

Nature: A pale green essence with the consistency of water or alcohol.

Odour description and effect: The aroma is delightfully citrus-like with just a hint of spice. Its effect is uplifting, antidepressant and refreshing.

Therapeutic uses: Colds and flu, fever, infectious illness, anxiety and depression.

Blends well with: Other citrus oils, basil, clary sage, lavender, neroli, cypress, geranium, juniper, coriander, ginger, frankincense, elemi.

Myth and magic: Bergamot is named after the Italian city of Bergamo in Lombardy. The oil was not known to the ancients. Its magical influence can be used to inspire peacefulness, happiness and pleasant dreams.

Price and availability: Medium price range; widely available.

CAUTIONS: Not to be used on skin shortly before exposure to sunlight as the oil is phototoxic and may cause brown blotching. While all citrus essences are potentially phototoxic, bergamot is the most hazardous in this respect. However, I have seen unsightly pigmentation occur when the oil was used prior to working in a hot and steamy hotel kitchen! Therefore, it may be best to use bergamot only as a room scent. However, it is possible to obtain bergamot FCF which is free of bergaptene (the substance which causes pigmentation to the skin). This variety of bergamot oil is safe to use on the skin at any time.

Lime
Citrus aurantifolia

Source: Expression of the peel of the unripe fruit from the small evergreen tree native to Asia. Most of the oil is produced in the USA and Italy. There is also a distilled oil of lime which is captured from the whole ripe crushed fruit. However, this has an inferior aroma, so always ask for the expressed oil.

Nature: A pale yellow or green liquid with the consistency of water or alcohol.

Odour description and effect: A sharp, fresh citrus scent. The odour effect is uplifting and refreshing.

Therapeutic uses: Cellulite, poor circulation, respiratory disorders, colds and flu, depression.

Blends well with: Other citrus oils, neroli, lavender, rosemary, clary sage, ylang ylang. Use only a tiny amount in blends as the aroma can be overpowering.

Myth and magic: Like lemon, lime can be used in self-purification rituals and to inspire peacefulness and happiness.

Price and availability: Lowest price range. Sometimes available from health shops and other retail outlets. More easily obtainable from specialist mail order suppliers.

CAUTIONS: Do not apply to the skin shortly before exposure to sunlight as it may cause brown blotching. Like most citrus oils, lime essence should be used in the very lowest concentrations, as it may cause irritation, especially to those with sensitive skin. This oil, like other citrus oils, has a short shelf-life so buy in small quantities and use within six to nine months.

Fragrant Earth

*These two heavy lingering essences impart a
'dark' quality to blends. Their rich earthy scents
engender a 'grounding' sensation.*

Patchouli
Pogostemon cablin

Source: Distillation of the dried and fermented leaves of the bushy plant native to tropical Asia. Most of the oil is produced in India, China, Malaysia and South America.

Nature: An amber, slightly viscous liquid.

Odour description and effect: A rich, earthy scent, becoming sweeter as it ages. Ideally, the oil needs to be at least two or three years old before the aroma is at its best. Its odour effect is warming and stimulating, though in tiny amounts (as a background to blends) it is a relaxant; a reputed aphrodisiac.

Therapeutic uses: Acne, athlete's foot, promotes growth of hair, dandruff, fungal infections, insect repellent, wounds, nervous exhaustion and stress-related complaints.

Blends well with: Cedarwood, lavender, rose, neroli, bergamot, clary sage, clove, geranium, vetiver, sandalwood.

Myth and magic: In magic, can be used to promote physical stamina and sexual potency.

Price and availability: Lowest price range; widely available.

Vetiver
Vetiveria zizanoides

Source: Distillation of the roots of the scented grass native to southern India, Indonesia and Sri Lanka. Most of the oil is obtained from cultivated plants grown in Réunion and the Comoro Islands.

Nature: A dark brown viscous liquid.

Odour description and effect: A rich earthy aroma with a molasses-like undertone. The fragrance improves as the oil ages. Its odour effect is calming and warming; a reputed aphrodisiac.

Therapeutic uses: Aching muscles, nervousness and tension, high blood pressure, insomnia, light-headedness, premenstrual syndrome, skin care.

Blends well with: Clary sage, citrus essences, sandalwood, geranium, rose, jasmine, patchouli, lavender, ylang ylang.

Myth and magic: Has been used in India for thousands of years for perfumery purposes. In magic, the oil is used to promote tranquillity and psychic protection.

Price and availability: Medium price range. Available from health shops and retail outlets.

A Touch Of Spice

The following essential oils are derived from spices which are very familiar in a culinary context. They are derived from seeds, buds, roots or bark of their particular plant.

Cardamom
Elettaria cardamom

Source: Distillation of the dried ripe fruit (seeds) of the reed-like herb native to Asia. Most of the oil is produced in India.

Nature: A colourless to pale yellow liquid with the consistency of water or alcohol.

Odour description and effect: A sweet-spicy, warming fragrance with a hint of eucalyptus. The odour effect is warming, head-clearing and stimulating; a reputed aphrodisiac.

Therapeutic uses: Digestive disturbances, mental fatigue, nervous exhaustion.

Blends well with: Cedarwood, frankincense, cinnamon, cloves, citrus essences, floral essences. Use in the lowest concentration as it has a high odour intensity which may overpower your blends.

Myth and magic: The ancient Egyptians used the seeds for medicinal purposes, while in India the seeds have been used for thousands of years for medicinal and culinary purposes and in the preparation of aphrodisiacal perfumes.

Price and availability: High price range. Available from health shops and retail outlets.

Cinnamon Bark
Cinnamomom zeylanicum

Source: Distillation of the bark chips from the small tree native to Sri Lanka, India and Madagascar. A lower grade oil is obtained from the leaves and twigs.

Nature: A light amber liquid with the consistency of water or alcohol.

Odour description and effect: A warm, spicy, dry, tenacious aroma. The effect is warming and stimulating; a reputed aphrodisiac.

Therapeutic uses: Used only in the vaporizer as an antidepressant room perfume, or as a fumigant during infectious illness.

Blends well with: Citrus essences, other spices, frankincense.

Myth and magic: A valued spice since ancient times. Brought to Europe by the Phoenicians.

Price and availability: Medium price range. Inferior cinnamon leaf oil is less expensive and widely available. Cinnamon bark oil is most easily available from mail order specialists.

CAUTIONS: A powerful skin irritant. Use only as a room scent.

Clove Bud
Eugenia caryophyllata

Source: Distillation of the buds of the slender evergreen tree native to Indonesia. Most of the oil is produced in Madagascar. A lower grade of clove oil with a less fruity aroma is distilled from the leaves and stems.

Nature: A light amber liquid with the consistency of water or alcohol.

Odour description and effect: A bitter-sweet, spicy aroma. The odour effect is warming and stimulating; a reputed aphrodisiac.

Therapeutic uses: Vaporized as a room scent, or used as a fumigant during infectious illness. Clove oil is used as a first-aid measure for toothache (while awaiting dental treatment).

Blends well with: Citrus essences, other spices, rose, vanilla, ylang ylang. Use in a very low concentration as the oil has a high odour intensity and may overpower your blends.

Myth and magic: The name is derived from the Latin *clavus* meaning 'nail', which the buds resemble. Cloves were one of the earliest spices mentioned in ancient Chinese writings.

Price and availability: Medium price range. Inferior clove leaf or stem oil is often available from retail outlets; however, clove bud oil is obtainable from mail order suppliers.

Black Pepper
Piper nigrum

Source: Distillation of the dried peppercorns of a woody vine native to south-west India. Most of the oil is produced in India; also distilled in Europe and the USA.

Nature: A pale greenish-yellow liquid with the consistency of water or alcohol.

Odour description and effect: A hot, spicy piquant odour. Its odour effect is stimulating and warming; a reputed aphrodisiac.

Therapeutic uses: Poor circulation, muscular aches and pains, loss of appetite, nausea, colds and flu, infections and viruses, lethargy and mental fatigue.

Blends well with: Other spices, citrus essences, jasmine, rose, lavender, ylang ylang, rosemary, sandalwood.

Myth and magic: In ancient times black pepper was very costly. For magical purposes, it can be used to stimulate conscious thought processes and to engender courage.

Price and availability: Medium price range. Available from health shops and retail outlets.

CAUTIONS: Use in the lowest concentration if you have sensitive skin

Coriander
Coriandrum sativum

Source: Distillation of the seeds (fruit) of the herb native to southern Europe and western Asia. Most of the oil is now produced in eastern Europe.

Nature: A colourless to pale yellow liquid with the consistency of water or alcohol.

Odour description and effect: A lighthearted fragrance with a sweet, spicy, faintly musky overtone. Its odour effect is warming, uplifting and stimulating; coriander was considered to be an aphrodisiac.

Therapeutic uses: Arthritis, muscular aches and pains, poor circulation, digestive problems, colds and flu, mental fatigue and nervous exhaustion.

Blends well with: Other spices, citrus essences, jasmine, frankincense, petitgrain, sandalwood, cypress, pine, juniper.

Myth and magic: Introduced to Europe by the Romans. During the Middle Ages it was used in love potions and to cure spots. For magical purposes, it can be used to stimulate mental clarity and to attract true love.

Price and availability: Medium price range, widely available.

Ginger
Zingiber officinale

Source: Distillation of the unpeeled, dried, ground root (rhizomes) of the plant native to southern Asia.

Nature: A pale yellow or amber liquid with the consistency of water or alcohol.

Odour description and effect: A warm, peppery-spicy scent, but not as pleasantly pungent as the fresh root. Sadly, the heat of distillation tends to distort the aroma. The odour effect is warming and stimulating; an aphrodisiac.

Therapeutic uses: Arthritis, muscular aches and pains, poor circulation, rheumatism, catarrh, coughs, sore throat, diarrhoea, colic, indigestion, nausea, travel sickness, colds and flu, debility, nervous exhaustion.

Blends well with: Coriander, citrus essences, sandalwood, vetiver, patchouli, frankincense, cedarwood, neroli, rose.

Myth and magic: Ginger has been cultivated for a very long time. It has been mentioned by Confucius and in the Koran. St Hildegarde, a twelfth-century healer, extolled the virtues of its aphrodisiacal properties, recommending it for older men married to energetic young women.

Price and availability: Medium price range. Sometimes available from retail outlets, more easily obtainable from mail order suppliers.

Juniper
Juniperus communis

Source: Distillation of the berries of the evergreen shrub native to the northern hemisphere. A lower grade oil with a harsh aroma is extracted from the needles and wood. Always use juniper berry oil.

Nature: A colourless liquid with the consistency of water or alcohol.

Odour description and effect: A fresh, woody aroma like pine but with a pleasant peppery kick. Its odour effect is warming, yet calming.

Therapeutic uses: Acne, eczema, haemorrhoids, oily skin conditions, cellulite, rheumatism, colds and flu, absence of periods outside pregnancy, cystitis, anxiety, nervous tension and stress-related problems.

Blends well with: Bergamot, elemi, cypress, rosemary, lavender, geranium, sandalwood.

Myth and magic: Has always been regarded as a magical plant and is used for protection.

Price and availability: Medium price range; superior berry oil from mail order suppliers.

CAUTIONS: Not to be used during pregnancy.

A Sensual Aromatherapy Selection

Although 39 oils are featured in Aphrodite's Pharmacy, you may find that just one or two essences will be enough to get you started on the fragrant path to sensual aromatherapy. However, if you intend to take the art of sensual aromatherapy seriously, you will probably need a basic selection of six or seven carefully chosen essences, enough to create a variety of fragrant accords.

Ideally, any initial selection of essences will include a representative from the floral, woody, citrus, spicy, resinous, herbaceous and earthy groups. But your final choice should be influenced by your personal preferences and those of your lover, and by price and availability of the oil. The panel below offers a few suggestions for your sensual aromatherapy selection kit.

Assembling Your Own Sensual Aromatherapy Kit

Aromatic box one
(inexpensive)
Geranium, petitgrain, grapefruit, coriander, elemi, lavender, patchouli

‗

Aromatic box two
(medium priced)
Ylang ylang, cedarwood, bergamot, black pepper, frankincense, lavender, patchouli

‗

Aromatic box three
(luxury selection)
Rose otto (or rose absolute), sandalwood, cardamom, jasmine, clary sage, vetiver

---

Do feel free to leave out a particular group of essences if the aromas do not generally appeal. Instead you could include more than one oil from a preferred group. However, bear in mind that an essence may smell unexciting on its own, but may take on an interesting persona once skilfully blended with other oils. For instance, many people find the rich, earthy aromas of vetiver and patchouli heavy-going as loners. Yet blend either of these oils with the lighter fragrances of bergamot, grapefruit or geranium, and there is a successful marriage of opposites. The bright citrus or floral essences act to awaken the senses, elevating the aroma to a higher plane. At the same time, the powerful embrace of vetiver or patchouli serves to hold back the more volatile essences whose presence would otherwise be relatively fleeting.

But what if your lover adores an aroma that you dislike? Before giving up on the oil, see what it smells like once it has merged with their natural body scent. Dilute one or two drops of the essential oil in a teaspoon of vegetable oil and rub into his or her forearm. Wait for at least half a minute for the odours to merge, then sniff. You may be pleasantly surprised. More often than not, the aromas we like best tend to blend harmoniously with our own unique essence.

Where to Buy Your Essential Oils

It is vital to obtain only the purest aromatherapy grade essential oils. Most aromatherapists obtain their oils from specialist mail order suppliers. Beginners can obtain good quality oils from many health shops or other retail outlets specializing in natural remedies. However, some shops sell oils labelled 'Aromatherapy oils', which means the bottles contain a mixture of about 2–3 per cent essential oil in a carrier such as almond oil. These are fine as massage oils, but such highly diluted blends cannot be used by the drop to perfume the bath water; neither are they suitable for use in vaporizers for perfuming rooms. As much as a tablespoon of an aromatherapy oil blend would be needed to perfume a bath or a room, whereas just four drops of pure essential oil is enough for the same purposes. Moreover, the shelf-life of diluted essential oils is drastically reduced.

Caring for Your Essential Oils

Essential oils can be damaged by exposure to light, extremes of temperature and prolonged exposure to oxygen in the air. For this reason they are sold in well-stoppered, dark glass bottles. In theory, most essential oils will keep for several years. However, with the exception of bergamot, citrus oils begin to deteriorate after about six months. A few oils improve with age, rather like some good wines. Examples of these are sandalwood, patchouli, frankincense and rose otto. But the more often you open the bottle, the greater the chance of oxidation and thus a lessening of the oil's therapeutic properties – as reflected in a deterioration of the aroma. Store your oils in a cool dark place and they will keep for at least a year. Once diluted in a base oil for massage, however, the blend will keep for no longer than two or three months.

Other Ambrosial Bounties

You may also find some or all of the following ingredients useful:

Floral waters: The hair tonics, cologne and aftershave blends suggested in the practical sections of this book are suspended in a base of rosewater, orange flower water, witch hazel or plain distilled water. Floral waters and distilled water are available from most pharmacies or herbal suppliers.

Whole spices: Some of the water-based room perfume formulas are prepared from whole spices such as cloves, ginger root, cinnamon stick, juniper berries and coriander. These are available from health shops, herbal suppliers, mail-order suppliers and good grocers.

Vanilla pod: As the solvent extracted oil of vanilla is so expensive and elusive, Chapter 9 includes a recipe for making your own infused oil of vanilla which can be used as a base for massage oil blends and perfume formulas.

Natural vanilla extract: This is vanilla suspended in alcohol, available from health shops and good supermarkets. It can be used in water-based room perfume blends.

Beeswax: Available from herbal suppliers, craft shops or from some bee-keepers. This is used as a base for the solid perfume formulas suggested in Chapter 9. Try to obtain honey-scented yellow beeswax rather than the refined white version.

Jojoba: An excellent carrier for perfume blends because it is virtually odourless and has a very long shelf-life. Available from most health shops or by mail-order from essential oil suppliers. The oil can be used for skin care.

Light coconut oil: A highly refined, virtually odourless oil with a very long shelf-life. An excellent base for perfume blends.

Almond oil: One of the finest base oils in which to dilute essential oils, especially for body massage. Other recommended base oils include sunflower or grapeseed. For facial treatments you may wish to use one of the more expensive vitamin-rich cold pressed oils such as avocado, peach kernel, extra virgin olive oil or hazelnut. These oils are available from health shops, some pharmacies or by mail order from essential oil suppliers.

(See the Appendix for further information on suppliers, further reading, equipment and measurements.)

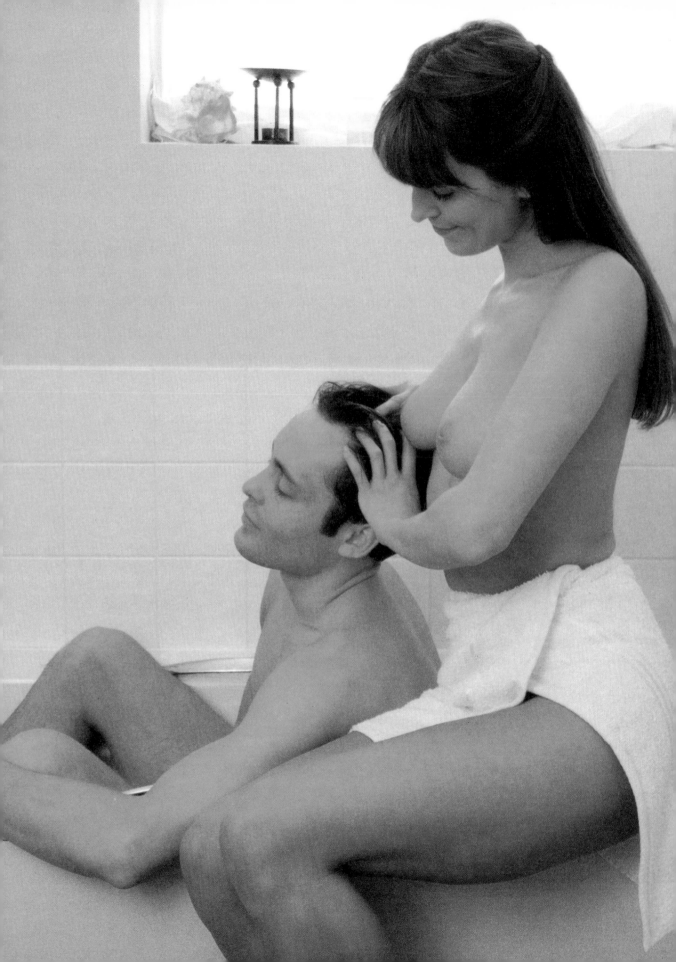

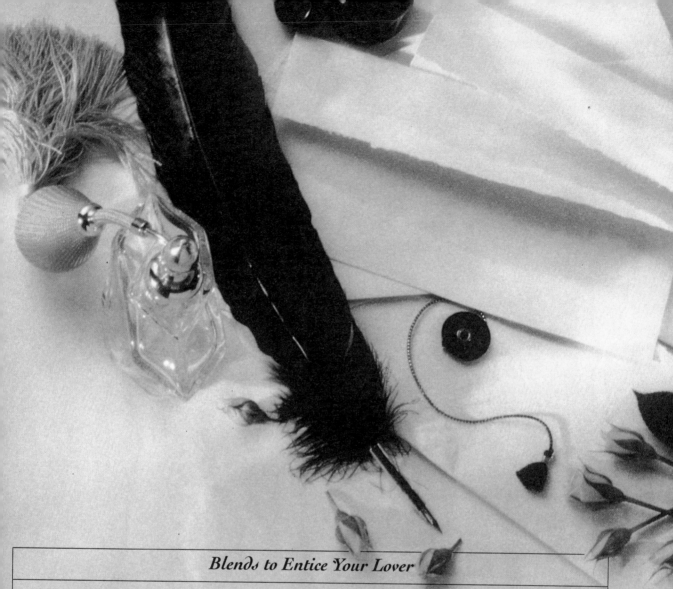

Blends to Entice Your Lover

Here are some blend suggestions to use on your scented love-note.
Simply mix together the oils – the recipes state the number of drops
of each to use – and you are ready to perfume the paper.

Lady Chatterley

OILS	DROPS
Bergamot	4
Coriander	1
Rose	1

Adonis

OILS	DROPS
Lemon	2
Rose	1
Sandalwood	2

Forever Scarlett

OILS	DROPS
Black pepper	2
Geranium	1
Ylang ylang	2

Truly, Madly, Deeply

OILS	DROPS
Bergamot	3
Clary sage	1
Grapefruit	1
Jasmine	1

Ode To Pan

OILS	DROPS
Cedarwood	2
Clary sage	1
Petitgrain	1
Vetiver	1

I Return

OILS	DROPS
Frankincense	1
Neroli	2
Orange	2

Mixing Massage Oils

In traditional aromatherapy, oils are chosen for specific conditions such as poor circulation, high blood pressure, muscular aches and pains and so on. Surprisingly, not all aromatherapists take the recipient's aroma preference into account. For erotic aromatherapy, however, the prime concern is to create a pleasing aromatic blend. You can choose to blend according to the top, middle and base note pattern if you wish, taking into account the aphrodisiac properties of the oils (*see page 59*). But the most important consideration is that both you and your partner find the aroma delightful. So always let your nose be your guide. However, if you are still unsure, try a few of the massage oil formulas suggested in Chapter 7.

Essential oils intended for massage need to be diluted in base oil at a rate of 0.5 to 3 per cent (*see opposite page*). The lowest concentrations (0.5 to 1 per cent) are best for facial oils and for those with sensitive skin. There are a number of base oils which are appropriate carrier oils for aromatherapy purposes (*see page 66 for more information on base oils*).

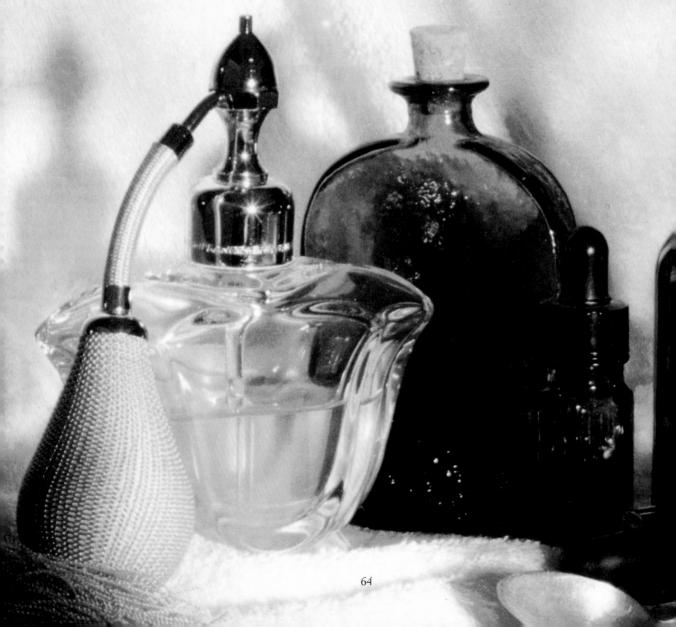

Important: Some oils have a high odour intensity and will overpower your blends unless used in quantities of 0.5 to 1 per cent. In the case of cardamom, even less than 0.5 per cent will often be sufficient. Other powerfully aromatic oils include: chamomile, jasmine, rose otto, peppermint and ginger.

The following essential oils should always be used in the lowest concentrations as well, because they are potential skin irritants. They include: basil, black pepper, ginger, grapefruit, jasmine, lemon, orange, peppermint and pine.

Easy Measures

For a full body massage you will need 30 ml of oil – more if the skin is dry or hairy. For a face massage, 5–10 ml will be sufficient. To mix small quantities of oil, use a 5 ml plastic medicine spoon (available from pharmacies) to measure the base oil. An ordinary teaspoon may hold less than 5 ml, but will suffice.

Blend Percentage	Essential Oil in Drops	Base Oil in Teaspoons
0.5	1	2
1	1	1
2	2	1
3	3	1

Blend Percentage	Essential Oil in Drops	Base Oil in Tablespoons
0.5	5	2
1	10	1
2	20	1
3	30	1

Base Oils

Essential oils intended for massage, and for other beauty and skin-care treatments, are diluted in a base oil or a floral water in some cases. This dilution is necessary since many essential oils will irritate the skin if applied directly (*see Before You Begin cautions, page 10*). The best base for aromatherapy purposes is an unrefined oil such as almond, olive, hazelnut or sunflower seed. Look for an oil that is labelled 'cold pressed' or 'unrefined'. Unlike refined oils such as soya or corn, unrefined oils are rich in fat-soluble nutrients and essential fatty acids which are excellent skin treatments in themselves. Extra-virgin olive-oil, for example, soothes inflamed skin. The oil has also been used for centuries as a beneficial rub for arthritic joints.

Never use mineral oil (baby oil) as this hinders the penetration of essential oils. It also tends to clog the pores of the skin thus contributing to the development of blackheads and pimples. Moreover, according to many health experts, mineral oil applied to the skin (or taken by mouth) makes fat-soluble nutrients such as vitamins A and E leach from the body.

Many aromatherapists favour bland base oils such as refined almond or grapeseed because such oils do not impart their own aroma to the fragrant blends. Yet to my nose the faintly nutty odour of unrefined vegetable oils (or its pungency, in the case of extra-virgin olive-oil), does, in fact, blend harmoniously with the aromas of essential oils. Moreover, unrefined base oils especially olive, impart their own sensual quality to the blend. Indeed, the ancient Greeks must have discovered this too, for this oil was sacred to Aphrodite, goddess of love, beauty and passion.

For a more economical, less nutty or pungent blend, you could mix a refined oil such as grapeseed with an equal quantity (or much less) of an unrefined oil such as hazelnut, extra-virgin olive or sunflower seed. If you use sesame oil, ensure that it is the light-coloured oil from the raw seed. The dark, strongly-flavoured oil obtained from the toasted seeds does not blend harmoniously with essential oils – unless you relish smelling like a stir-fry! Dark sesame oil may also cause skin irritation in some people.

For a facial oil, jojoba (pronounced ho-ho-ba) is one of the lightest to use, either alone or mixed with other vegetable oils. It can even be used on oily or acneous skin, as a carrier for the essential oils. In fact, jojoba is a liquid wax rather than a true vegetable oil. It is extracted from the seeds of a small evergreen plant native to the desert regions of Mexico, Arizona and California.

Other beneficial oils especially suitable for facial treatment are avocado, peachnut, apricot kernel, passion-flower and evening primrose. Although avocado is one of the richest oils, it is highly penetrative, and makes an excellent treatment for dry skin. It can be mixed half-and-half with a lighter oil such as almond, apricot kernel or peachnut.

Evening primrose oil is especially helpful in preventing vital moisture loss from the skin, and passion-flower oil is believed to help maintain skin elasticity. Both these oils are usually taken by mouth (in capsule form) for maintaining skin health. However, you can add the contents of a capsule to your facial oil formulas (1 capsule to every 2 or 3 teaspoons of another base oil). But do remember to use these blends within a few weeks, for these two oils have a short shelf-life.

High quality vegetable oils suitable for aromatherapy are widely available from good supermarkets and delicatessens. Speciality oils such as apricot kernel, almond, evening primrose, jojoba and avocado are to be found in many health shops and pharmacies.

Essential Oils and Beauty Care

Care of the skin needs to go deeper than superficial 'beauty care' and it need not be an exclusively female activity, as the word 'beauty' implies. In fact, a healthy skin is an accurate barometer of emotional and physical harmony, and indeed, disharmony. So no amount of external treatment will help much if you exist on a junk food diet, have a frenzied lifestyle with little or no time to relax, and if your emotions are generally out of balance. First treat your skin from this perspective and the oils will work more efficiently, adding much more than just a seductive sheen!

In simple terms, skin is far more than just a covering for the body; it is a living, breathing organism. It has a two-way job; firstly, protecting the body from infection and dirt, and secondly, eliminating toxins. If the body is healthy, skin cell regeneration goes on unceasingly.

Skin health is also affected by genetics, age, environment, attention – or lack of it. Even if you are one of the lucky few, blessed with a fine trouble-free skin, the use of the finest vegetable oils and essences will not only help to preserve its suppleness for as long as possible, but will improve your health in general. As we have already seen, essential oils applied to the skin (and inhaled) reach the bloodstream and lymph system from where they continue to exert their therapeutic effect.

Many essential oils help to balance sebum (the skin's natural oil secretion which acts to slow down the evaporation of moisture), and to generally tone the complexion by supporting capillary function.

How to Use Essential Oils in Skin-care

First choose the appropriate essence(s) for your skin type (*refer to the Skin-care Chart on page 68*), taking into account your aroma preferences. Then prepare a massage oil blend as described on page 64. Do not forget to make a separate, low concentration mixture of oils for the more sensitive skin of the face. There are three different ways of applying oils for skin treatments.

Method 1: Apply a fine film of your blend just after a bath or shower when your skin is still warm and moist. The oils will penetrate the skin within twenty or thirty minutes. So, unless you have applied too much oil, there should be no need to wipe off any excess.

Method 2: Apply after a deep cleansing facial sauna or steam bath. Facial saunas are good for city skins or for those times when you feel your skin needs a pick-me-up or to quell an eruption of spots. Skin eruptions are common to many of us in times of stress and in women during the premenstrual phase. Avoid steam treatments if you have thread veins – the heat will dilate the blood vessels, thus worsening the condition. Also avoid if you have asthma, since concentrated steam can trigger an attack.

To make a facial sauna, simply shake one or two drops of a suitable essential oil for your skin type into a bowl containing 0.5 litres of steaming water. Cover your whole head with a towel and put it over the steaming bowl so the towel forms a tent to catch the vapour. Stay there for up to five minutes. Finish the treatment by splashing your face with cold water to remove wastes accumulated on the surface of the skin. Wait about fifteen minutes for your skin to settle down, then apply your chosen aromatic oil treatment.

Method 3: Apply shortly before going for a walk in the open air (preferably the park or unpolluted country air). The combination of oxygen and essential oil is a superb and natural skin rejuvenator.

Skin-care Chart – Essential and Base Oils

Skin type	Essential oils	Base oils
Normal	Chamomile, geranium, lavender, neroli, rose otto	Almond, apricot kernel, extra-virgin olive, peachnut, sunflower seed
Dry	Lavender, neroli, rose otto, sandalwood	Almond, avocado, evening primrose (1 capsule to every 10 ml of another base oil), extra-virgin olive, peachnut, sunflower seed
Oily	Bergamot FCF, cypress, frankincense, geranium, lavender, rosemary	Hazelnut, jojoba **Important:** Apply after a bath or shower for maximum penetration
Combination	Chamomile, geranium, lavender, rose otto	Extra-virgin olive, hazelnut, jojoba, peachnut
Sensitive	Chamomile, neroli or lavender	Apricot kernel, jojoba
Acne	Frankincense, juniper, lavender, patchouli, sandalwood	Jojoba **Important:** Apply after bath or shower to facilitate maximum penetration. Do not remove excess
Puffy	Cypress, geranium, lavender, patchouli	Almond, extra-virgin olive, sunflower seed
Thread veins	Chamomile, neroli, rose otto	Apricot kernel, extra-virgin olive, jojoba, peachnut
Ageing	Frankincense, geranium, rose otto, sandalwood	Apricot kernel, avocado, extra-virgin olive, passion-flower (contents of 1 capsule to every 10 ml of another base oil), peachnut, sunflower seed

Skin-care Chart – Blends for Specific Skin Types

Skin type	OIL	AMOUNT	OIL	AMOUNT	OIL	AMOUNT
Normal	Chamomile	1 drop	Chamomile	2 drops	Geranium	1 drop
	Geranium	2 drops	Rose otto	2 drops	Lavender	2 drops
	Lavender	2 drops	Apricot kernel	25 ml	Neroli	2 drops
	Almond	15 ml			Almond	20 ml
	Sunflower seed	10 ml			Extra-virgin olive	5 ml
Dry	Sandalwood	5 drops	Lavender	3 drops	Lavender	3 drops
	Sunflower seed	20 ml	Rose otto	1 drop	Neroli	2 drops
	Avocado	5 ml	Almond	20 ml	Extra-virgin olive	5 ml
			Evening primrose	2 caps	Peachnut	20 ml
Oily	Frankincense	2 drops	Cypress	2 drops	Bergamot FCF	2 drops
	Lavender	3 drops	Geranium	2 drops	Rosemary	3 drops
	Jojoba	25 ml	Lavender	1 drop	Hazelnut	10 ml
			Hazelnut	25 ml	Jojoba	15 ml
Combination	Chamomile	2 drops	Chamomile	1 drop	Geranium	2 drops
	Rose otto	1 drop	Geranium	1 drop	Lavender	3 drops
	Peachnut	25 ml	Lavender	3 drops	Hazelnut	5 ml
			Extra-virgin olive	10 ml	Peachnut	20 ml
			Jojoba	15 ml		
Sensitive	Chamomile	2 drops	Neroli	2 drops	Lavender	3 drops
	Apricot kernel	20 ml	Jojoba	20 ml	Apricot kernel	10 ml
					Jojoba	10 ml
Acne	Frankincense	1 drop	Juniper	2 drops	Juniper	3 drops
	Lavender	3 drops	Sandalwood	3 drops	Lavender	2 drops
	Patchouli	1 drop	Jojoba	25 ml	Jojoba	25 ml
	Jojoba	25 ml				
Puffy	Cypress	3 drops	Geranium	3 drops	Cypress	2 drops
	Geranium	2 drops	Patchouli	2 drops	Geranium	1 drop
	Almond oil	20 ml	Extra-virgin olive	5 ml	Lavender	2 drops
	Extra-virgin olive	5 ml	Sunflower seed	20 ml	Almond	25 ml
Thread veins	Chamomile	1 drop	Chamomile	2 drops	Neroli	3 drops
	Neroli	1 drop	Neroli	2 drops	Rose otto	1 drop
	Rose otto	1 drop	Peachnut	25 ml	Apricot kernel	25 ml
	Extra-virgin olive	5 ml				
	Jojoba oil	20 ml				
Ageing	Frankincense	1 drop	Sandalwood	5 drops	Frankincense	2 drops
	Rose otto	1 drop	Sunflower seed	15 ml	Geranium	3 drops
	Sandalwood	2 drops	Avocado	10 ml	Apricot kernel	15 ml
	Passion-flower	2 capsules			Extra-virgin olive	10 ml
	Peachnut	20 ml				

Oils for Hair and Scalp

The finest vegetable oil for the hair is extra-virgin olive, which is known to strengthen the hair shafts, thus giving the hair body and shine. Castor oil, extracted from the seeds of the attractive castor oil shrub, was used in the past as a hair thickener. It is a wonderful hair shiner and despite being a very sticky oil, it is surprisingly easy to wash out. Another excellent hair and scalp oil is peachnut. Because it is much lighter than olive-oil, it is suitable for most hair and scalp conditions, except the very oily. In this instance, a water-based hair tonic would be preferable (*see opposite page*).

How to Make a Hair and Scalp Oil

First choose the essential oil most suitable for your hair and scalp condition, taking into account your aroma preference (*see chart below*). Add up to 20 drops to a 50 ml bottle of base oil and shake well.

Hair and Scalp Chart – Oils and Oil Formulas

Hair type	Essential oils	Base oils	Suggested hair oil formula	
			OIL	AMOUNT
Normal	Geranium, lavender, mandarin, rose otto	Extra-virgin olive, jojoba, peachnut	Geranium Lavender Mandarin Extra-virgin olive	5 drops 5 drops 5 drops 50 ml
Dry	Chamomile, lavender, sandalwood, ylang ylang	Extra-virgin olive, peachnut, sunflower seed	Sandalwood Ylang ylang Extra-virgin olive Peachnut	15 drops 5 drops 25 ml 25 ml
Oily	Bergamot FCF, cypress, frankincense, lavender, rosemary			
Dandruff (Dry scalp)	Chamomile, geranium, lavender	Extra-virgin olive	Chamomile Geranium Extra-virgin olive	5 drops 15 drops 50 ml
Dandruff (Oily scalp)	Cypress, cedarwood, patchouli, rosemary			
Healthy growth	Rosemary, patchouli, ylang ylang	Extra-virgin olive, castor (not for oily hair)	Patchouli Ylang ylang Castor Extra-virgin olive	10 drops 10 drops 25 ml 25 ml

Apply to wet hair (otherwise it will be difficult to shampoo out), then cover your head with a towel and leave for fifteen to thirty minutes before shampooing. Use your essential oil hair blend as a weekly conditioning treatment.

Aromatic Hair Tonics

These are massaged into the scalp several times a week. If used regularly they will improve the condition of your hair as well as making it smell good. Because they use waters, distill and floral, rather than oils as a base, there is no need to wet your hair before applying.

Choose an appropriate essential oil for your hair and scalp condition, taking into account your aroma preference. Add up to 15 drops of essential oil to 300 ml of a hair tonic base (*see charts on this and the previous page*). Remember to shake the bottle each time before use to disperse the essential oils.

Hair and Scalp Chart – Hair Tonics

Hair type	Tonic base	Suggested tonic formula OIL/TONIC BASE	AMOUNT
Normal	Distilled water, orange flower water, or a 50/50 mixture of distilled water and orange flower water	Geranium Lavender Orange flower water	3 drops 10 drops 300 ml
Dry	Distilled water, rosewater, or a 50/50 mixture of distilled water and rosewater.	Sandalwood Ylang ylang Rosewater	8 drops 5 drops 300 ml
Oily	A 50/50 mixture of distilled water and witch hazel, or a 50/50 mixture of distilled water and orange flower water, or a 50/50 mixture of distilled water and rosewater	Bergamot FCF Frankincense Rosemary Distilled water Witch hazel	5 drops 3 drops 5 drops 150 ml 150 ml
Dandruff (Dry scalp)	Distilled water or a 50/50 mixture of distilled water and rosewater	Geranium Lavender Distilled water	5 drops 10 drops 300 ml
Dandruff (Oily scalp)	A 50/50 mixture of witch hazel and distilled water, or a 50/50 mixture of witch hazel and orange flower water, or a 50/50 mixture of witch hazel and rosewater	Cedarwood Rosemary Distilled water Witch hazel	5 drops 10 drops 150 ml 150 ml
Healthy growth	Distilled water, or according to scalp condition (see 'normal', 'dry', 'oily', 'dandruff')	**Normal to oily:** rosemary distilled water **Normal to dry:** ylang ylang distilled water	15 drops 300 ml 15 drops 300 ml

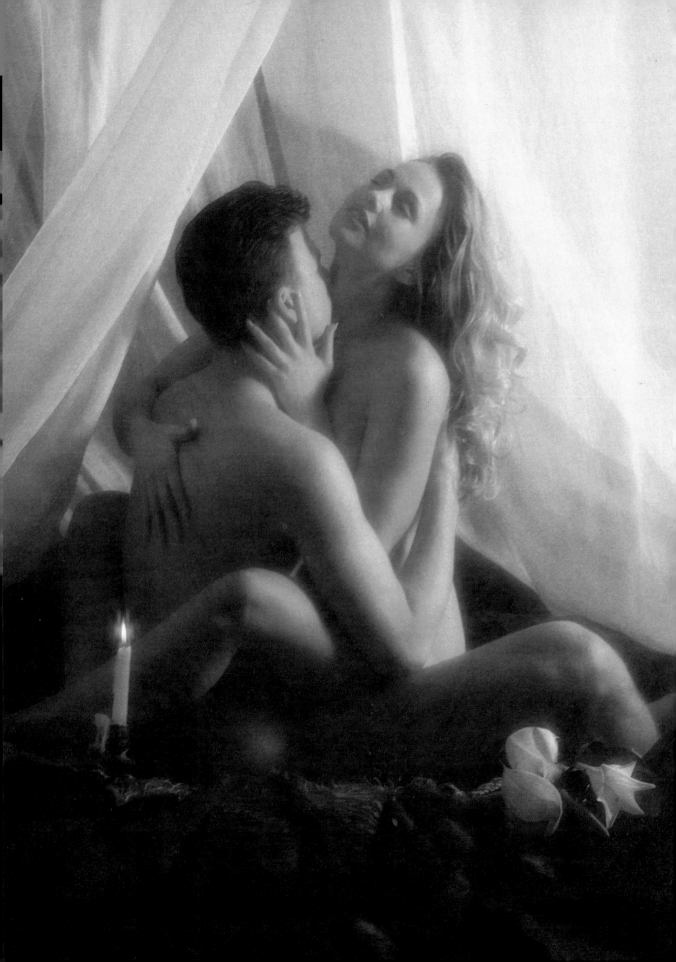

CHAPTER 5

Ambience of Enchantment

*... the outer room, balmy with rich perfumes,
should contain a bed, soft, agreeable to the sight,
covered with a clean white cloth, low in the middle part,
having garlands and bunches of flowers upon it,
and a canopy above it, and two pillows,
one at the top, another at the bottom.
There should be a sort of couch besides
and at the head of this a sort of stool, on which
should be placed the fragrant ointments for the night,
as well as flowers ... and other fragrant substances.*

The Kama Sutra

Setting the Scene

Having invited your lover to spend some fragrant moments with you, it is important to set the scene, which can be as simple or as elaborate as you like. Simply clear the room of any clutter, unplug the phone, dim the lights, prepare the oils – and let your imagination do the rest. However, by far the most magical way is to work together, to regard the act of preparation as a sort of ritual, a prelude to the special moment you are about to share. In so doing you will impart a romantic and spiritual quality to your lovemaking.

Although most people will choose the bedroom for their magical space, any other room can be elevated to a higher plane, especially if it has an open fire. Albeit a luxury available to few, what form of heating could be more seductive than a log fire? But even if you have to rely on a radiator or a portable gas fire for warmth, the skilful use of colour, lighting, music, plants and fragrance will merge into a harmonious whole, transforming the humblest of rooms into a garden of enchantment.

Colour and Lighting

Ideally, the room you choose will be decorated in soft hues rather than harsh avant-garde colour clashes such as bright orange with scarlet, or salmon pink and yellow – or even worse, vermilion with black zigzags! According to colour therapists, such inharmonious colour mixes can have a significant cumulative effect on mood and behaviour, exacerbating any existing feelings of stress or nervous tension. On the other hand, too much black, grey or dark brown can contribute to a depressive outlook – whether used to decorate a room or worn as clothing. Bright or clear colours have the opposite effect, contributing to a sense of well-being – just like a warm summer's day. It is also important to know that while red can be sexually stimulating under some conditions, too much red can be oppressive for some people.

However, there is no need to paint or wallpaper a room specially for the purpose of creating an erotic sanctuary. As long as the basic decor is gentle, the easiest and most economical way to tint the atmosphere is through lighting. A coloured light-bulb (preferably in a table lamp rather than the central light fitting), can be highly effective. But do bear in mind that a cold blue or green light is hardly conducive to passion. On the other hand, red light tends to mask all the other hues in a room. Far better to choose a subtle pink or peach light-bulb. Alternatively, drape a coloured shawl or silk scarf over a lampshade – but do ensure the material is not in direct contact with the bulb. Apart from the risk of scorching or burning a hole in the beautiful fabric, this could be a dangerous fire risk.

But surely the most romantic light must be the warm, flickering glow of candles. Put them in attractive candle holders, or use floating candles. If you do use floating candles, you might like to add some red or pink rose petals, or several heads of tiny flowers (if in season), to the bowl of water containing the candle.

Music

Music has the power to intensify our feelings, to evoke images and memories and to transport us into a state of exhilaration or melancholy, or simply to charm us through the delicacy of melody. In tribal dance rituals, frantic monotonous drumming and synchronized movement can lead to a state of trance or even ecstasy, while the drones and chants of Tibetan monks brings about a state of inner peace and unity.

Even though scientists are at a loss to explain exactly how music, singing and chanting influence our state of consciousness, we do know that a sense of rhythm and timing is inherent to human nature. Music therapists have found that musical rhythm with a rate of less than eighty beats per minute is perceived as 'slow', and so tends to relax and soothe; whereas more than ninety beats per minute is 'fast', and so exhilarates and excites. Indeed, every music lover has experienced the sensation of altered rate and rhythm of pulse and breathing – and the associated mood change. But just like our responses to fragrance, the specific thoughts and feelings evoked vary in proportion and intensity according to the nature of the sound and the ideas already in the mind. For this reason, it is difficult to suggest a list of mood-enhancing music suitable for everyone.

So when choosing music for your erotic sanctuary, think of the songs or melodies that are especially evocative of peak moments in your relationship – almost all lovers have their special music. However, while this can be played before, during and after lovemaking, it may not be suitable for giving erotic massage (*see page 98*).

As you will discover, in order to build up an erotic charge, sensual massage needs to be performed with slow, smooth and flowing movements. Likewise, the most appropriate music for massage is flowing and rhythmic, not loud, erratic or jerky. This is because it is virtually impossible to stop yourself moving in time with the music. Imagine then what it would be like to be massaged to the sounds of a heavy metal piece, or to the *1812 Overture*, cannon fire and all. Good fun for a few maybe, but nerve wracking or exhausting for lesser mortals.

A Bed of Fragrance

The Romans were obsessed with scent, especially the exquisite perfume of rose. At debauched banquets in honour of Bacchus, god of wine, roses were strewn everywhere; even the cushions and mattresses were stuffed with petals. As well as being regarded as a powerful aphrodisiac, its scent was believed to quell the intoxicating effects of alcohol, which meant they could drink more. The Roman emperor Nero is reputed to have slept on a bed of rose petals, an indulgence he probably gleaned from Cleopatra's seduction of Mark Antony.

Napoleon and Josephine indulged in scented pillow fights (well, metaphorically speaking at least), he delighted in a bedroom perfumed with rosemary cologne and she, the animal scent of musk oil. Napolean detested the odour of musk, but Josephine, being a hot-blooded Creole, was reluctant to conform to her lover's insipid European taste. That is, until he happened upon a bottle of Egyptian jasmine oil which he gave his beloved as a present. From then on their lovemaking must have been elevated to another dimension.

Many aromatic plants have been used as 'sleeping love charms'. This is an old English charm to ensure that you will dream of your true love and will marry within the year. At dawn on Midsummer's eve, gather a sprig of St John's wort with the dew still on it. Pass it through the smoke of the Midsummer bonfire. The same evening, place it under your pillow and your true love will appear in a dream

Today's lovers can enjoy a subtly perfumed bed by covering it with a pair of scented sheets. Choose any colour, although carefully ironed, white linen is very romantic, especially on sultry summer nights. To perfume sheets (and pillow-cases if you like) add up to 6 drops of essential oil to every 50 ml of water in a perfume atomizer or plant-mister and spray the sheets with a fine mist. Leave to dry before putting on the bed. It would be a good idea to use a different fragrance from that which you intend to use for the massage or as a room perfume. This will keep the sense of smell acute. Even though the nose quickly tires in the presence of the same fragrance, it can be awakened by a new aroma. Use an enlivening essence such as rosemary or lemon, the refreshing scent of lavender, geranium or bergamot, the cooling fragrances of cypress, pine or juniper.

The Language Of Flowers

Flowers, of course, are a must for your magical space. According to the 'language of flowers', whose origins can be traced back to ancient Turkey, flowers communicate to the hearts of lovers. This silent language reached its climax in Victorian times, capturing the imagination on a grand scale. In an age when chaperones were compulsory for ladies, it was intriguing for lovers to send coded messages to each other. Yet with the passage of time, it is only the red rose whose sweet mellow voice can still be heard. Indeed, few lovers of any culture would be at a loss to understand her *code de l'amour*. But let's give other flowers a chance to have their say, in the hope that it will help to revive this charming language.

Nowhere has the language of flowers been expressed more erotically than in D. H. Lawrence's *Lady Chatterley's Lover*. The following passage is a wonderful example of Lawrence's gift with this most beguiling of languages.

The rain had ceased. There was a wet, heavy, perfumed stillness. ... And when he came near, his eyes looked into hers, but she could not understand the meaning. He had brought columbines and campions, and new-mown hay, and oak-tufts and honeysuckle in small bud. He fastened fluffy young oak-sprays round her breasts, sticking in tufts of bluebells and campion: and in her navel he poised a pink campion flower, and in her maiden-hair were forget-me-nots and woodruff.

Living Fragrance

You may wish to perfume your magical space with fragrant plants instead of essential oils. The rose is an obvious first choice for lovers; but not all roses are fragrant. The oldest known rose and the most beautifully scented is Rosa gallica, sometimes known as Rosa rubra, the classic red rose which was grown in temple gardens in ancient Persia in 1200 BC. Then there is the damask rose, Rosa damascena, a decendant of R. gallica; it is small and elegant, often with deep pink blooms and a delicious rich scent. There are, of course, many other scented roses in a myriad of colours, so you are sure to find a rose that is especially appealing.

But there are other flowers which can be cut and used to perfume your magical space, including: lavender, lemon balm, lemon verbena, brunfelsia, honeysuckle, jonquil, narcissus, lilac, mignonette, carnation, heliotrope, pink, night-scented stock, hyacinth, sweet pea, sweet William, violet, wallflower, jasmine, gardenia and lemon-scented geranium. Several of these flowers can be grown in pots indoors, but if you do not have a garden in which to grow any of the others, most will be available from good florists.

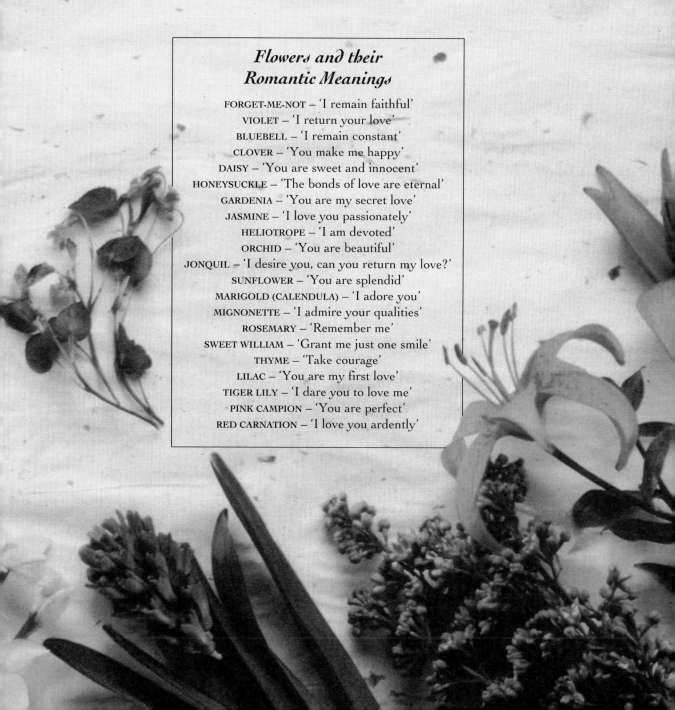

Flowers and their Romantic Meanings

FORGET-ME-NOT – 'I remain faithful'
VIOLET – 'I return your love'
BLUEBELL – 'I remain constant'
CLOVER – 'You make me happy'
DAISY – 'You are sweet and innocent'
HONEYSUCKLE – 'The bonds of love are eternal'
GARDENIA – 'You are my secret love'
JASMINE – 'I love you passionately'
HELIOTROPE – 'I am devoted'
ORCHID – 'You are beautiful'
JONQUIL – 'I desire you, can you return my love?'
SUNFLOWER – 'You are splendid'
MARIGOLD (CALENDULA) – 'I adore you'
MIGNONETTE – 'I admire your qualities'
ROSEMARY – 'Remember me'
SWEET WILLIAM – 'Grant me just one smile'
THYME – 'Take courage'
LILAC – 'You are my first love'
TIGER LILY – 'I dare you to love me'
PINK CAMPION – 'You are perfect'
RED CARNATION – 'I love you ardently'

Scenting the Room

There are several methods for perfuming rooms, although some are more effective and longer-lasting than others. The simplest is to add a few drops of essential oil to the water of a plant-mister or perfume atomizer. Add between 5 and 10 drops of your chosen essence(s) to 140 ml of water and shake well before each use. However, do not spray near highly polished wooden furniture since some essential oils dissolve varnish. Despite this alarming fact, they are kind to living tissue. The only drawback with room sprays is that the effect is so short-lived.

If you have a radiator humidifier, up to 10 drops of essential oil can be added to the water. This is a good method to use during cool weather when the central heating is on. The problem with some humidifiers, however, is that the water does not get warm enough to effectively diffuse the essential oils.

Another simple method is to put 1 or 2 drops on a cold light-bulb. Switch on the light and *voilà* – a scented room. But the aroma rarely lasts for longer than twenty minutes, especially if you use the highly volatile citrus oils. Moreover, with continual use, the light-bulb eventually becomes sticky and discoloured.

It is possible to buy a fragrance ring, a disc made either of ceramic or cardboard that balances over the top of a light-bulb. The essences are dropped on the ring and the warmth from the bulb releases the aromatic vapour. This is fine in theory; in practice the ring soon becomes very sticky, attracting tiny flies which seem to die on contact with the oils – a very unattractive sight!

By far the most effective way to perfume a room is to use a purpose-designed essential oil vaporizer – either an electric diffuser which usually vaporizes neat essences or a night-light candle burner which has a reservoir for water, to which you may add your essential oils.

Electric Diffusers

These gadgets are the high-tech alternative to candles and night-light vaporizers. A few drops of essential oil is dropped directly on to the ceramic or filter surface which is kept at a constant warm temperature. There is just enough heat to release the fragrance without risk of burning. However, the drawback with a number of electric fragrancers is that they cannot take water-based blends. You will have to forgo the pleasures of vaporizing your own water-based room perfumes made from whole spices

Blending for the Electric Diffuser

If you have chosen the type of electric vaporizer which cannot take oils suspended in water, you will need to use about 3 or 4 drops of neat essential oil to perfume an average-sized room. If you have found a complex blend that you particularly like, you could mix several undiluted essences together in a little bottle, using just a few drops of the blend on the ceramic or filter surface. If you use more than 6 drops of essential oil in an electric diffuser, the aroma can be overpowering.

The Night-light Vaporizer

By far the most effective way to perfume a room is to use a nightlight vaporizer or 'burner' as they are often called. Many of the burners are attractive to look at, and are usually made with materials such as earthenware (sometimes glass, porcelain or marble), with petal-shaped openings cut out of the sides to afford a free flow of air for the night-light candle which is placed inside. A small, sometimes detachable reservoir fits over the night-light and is filled with water. A few drops of essential oil is then floated on the surface and this is gently heated by the flame. As the aromatic water evaporates, the room becomes permeated with fragrance. If burned in a dimly lit or darkened room, and if there is a slight breeze, floral patterns dance on the wall like shadow puppets. The elements of earth (the clay), fire (the flame), water and air (the aromatic vapour) combine to create a magical effect.

However, if you forget to refill the reservoir after the water has evaporated, you may be left with a sticky, blackened residue of burned oil. This can be difficult to remove, unless you use an alcohol-based substance such as surgical spirit. One way to reduce the possibility of this happening is to buy a vaporizer with a reservoir deep enough to hold about 30 ml of water. This should vaporize for a few hours before needing to be refilled. Despite the drawbacks of having to keep an eye on this type of essential oil vaporizer, to my mind, the price of taking a little extra care is well worth the reward – an ambience of enchantment.

Blending for the Night-light Vaporizer

Fill the reservoir with water, then float 4 to 6 drops of essential oil on the water. For complex blends you may prefer to make an aromatic water. Simply mix 15 to 20 drops of essential oil to a 100–125ml bottle of water, then fill the reservoir with some of the blend. But do remember to shake the bottle each time before use to facilitate the complete dispersal of the oil in the water.

You might like to mix the essential oils with rosewater or orange flower water. Both blend exceptionally well with floral or citrus essences or with tiny quantities of spice oils. Or you could vaporize an aromatic decoction (prepared from whole spices) with the addition of essential oils if desired (*see the following page for aromatic decoctions*).

Essential Oil-based Room Perfume Blends

The following essential oil blends can be added to a water-filled vaporizer, radiator humidifier, the molten wax of a candle or the ceramic dish or filter-surface of an electric diffuser. Essential oil quantities are given in drops:

Dreamtime

OIL	DROPS
Chamomile	2
Lavender	2
Neroli	2

Siren

OIL	DROPS
Neroli	2
Rose	2
Ylang ylang	2

Spicy Moments

OIL	DROPS
Bergamot	4
Cardamom	1
Clove	1

Pagan

OIL	DROPS
Cedarwood	1
Pine	3
Rosemary	2

Dream Blossom

OIL	DROPS
Chamomile	2
Petitgrain	2
Rose	2

Enchantment

OIL	DROPS
Geranium	2
Orange	2
Ylang ylang	2

Eastern Promise

OIL	DROPS
Coriander	2
Frankincense	2
Ginger	1

Intrigue

OIL	DROPS
Elemi	1
Juniper	3
Vetiver	1

Dreams of Desire

OIL	DROPS
Juniper	2
Mandarin	2
Vetiver	1

Embrace

OIL	DROPS
Bergamot	2
Jasmine	2
Sandalwood	2

Firebird

OIL	DROPS
Cinnamon bark	1
Orange	3
Ylang ylang	2

Earth Magic

OIL	DROPS
Cypress	3
Frankincense	2
Petitgrain	2

Aromatic Decoctions

A decoction is an aqueous extraction of hard or woody plant material. You can use an aromatic decoction in a night-light vaporizer to perfume your magical space.

Choose highly aromatic plant material such as whole cloves, dried ginger root, a cinnamon stick, allspice berries, cardamom seeds, coriander seeds or a vanilla pod. If strong enough, a spicy decoction can be vaporized just as it is, or it can be made more aromatic with the addition of a few drops of essential oil. Spicy decoctions also smell wonderful blended 50/50 with orange flower water or rosewater.

Basic Method for Making a Decoction

You will need approximately 2 rounded teaspoons of dried plant material (e.g. coriander seed, allspice berries, whole cloves) to half a pint (240 ml) of water.

1 If possible, roughly grind the spices (except cloves) in a pestle and mortar, coffee grinder, or food processor for a few seconds to help release their volatile oils.

2 Put the plant material and water into a small stainless steel, enamel or pyrex saucepan with a tight fitting lid. Do not use an aluminium vessel as the metal may react with the spices, spoiling the aroma.

3 Bring the mixture to the boil and simmer for no more than five minutes, otherwise the decoction will boil away.

4 Turn off the heat, leave tightly covered and allow the decoction to stand for at least eight hours or overnight.

5 When ready, pour the decoction through fine muslin or a fine mesh tea strainer, then funnel into a glass bottle. Store in the fridge, but use within one or two months. If you intend to keep the decoction for longer, add a tablespoon of high proof, odourless vodka to the blend. This will extend the shelf-life for at least another month.

Other plant materials can be used to make decoctions and may be prepared as follows:

Ginger root: Bruise a dried root by hitting with a wooden mallet or the end of a rolling pin before proceeding as above.

Cinnamon stick: A quarter of a stick will be enough for 240 ml of water.

Nutmeg: Grate a quarter of a whole nutmeg into 240 ml of water.

Vanilla pod: Split down the middle, then cut into small pieces. Proceed with the basic method. Alternatively, you could use natural vanilla extract which is available from health shops and good supermarkets. Add 1 teaspoon of vanilla to every 50 ml of water. (*To make infused oil of vanilla to use as a perfume or massage oil base, see page 147.*)

You can make your own concentrated vanilla extract by simply splitting the vanilla pod lengthwise, then putting it into a glass jar or jug and covering with 50 ml of vodka. Cover the jar and allow to steep for at least six weeks. Even when ready to use (as a flavouring for desserts, or for use in a nightlight vaporizer, leave the vanilla pod in the vodka. The mixture will continue to strengthen, which means you can add a little more vodka if you wish.

On the opposite page are a number of water-based room perfume blends which use decoctions and floral waters in combination with essential oils. These water-based perfume blends can be used in your night-light vaporizer to create hours of fragrance.

Water-based Room Perfume Blends

The following water-based room perfume blends can be added to a water-filled vaporizer, radiator humidifier or the reservoir of a night-light vaporizer. Essential oil quantities are given in drops while decoction quantities are measured in millilitres.

Whispers of Spice

OIL/BASE	AMOUNT
Allspice decoction	50 ml
Orange flower water	50 ml

Fiery Lady

OIL/BASE	AMOUNT
Cinnamon decoction,	25 ml
Clove decoction	25 ml
Orange flower water	50 ml

Rose of India

OIL/BASE	AMOUNT
Cardamom decoction	50 ml
Rosewater	50 ml

Sunlight of the Grove

OIL/BASE	AMOUNT
Grapefruit	2 drops
Mandarin	4 drops
Nutmeg decoction	50 ml
Orange flower water	50 ml

Joi de Vivre

OIL/BASE	AMOUNT
Lemon	4 drops
Orange	4 drops
Ginger decoction	100 ml

Fruits of Love

OIL/BASE	AMOUNT
Bergamot	2 drops
Orange	2 drops
Petitgrain	2 drops
Coriander decoction	100 ml

Sweet Rapture

OIL/BASE	AMOUNT
Geranium	2 drops
Grapefruit	3 drops
Lavender	3 drops
Clove decoction	50 ml
Coriander decoction	50 ml

Interlude

OIL/BASE	AMOUNT
Bergamot	3 drops
Lavender	4 drops
Clove decoction	100 ml

Ode to Passion

OIL/BASE	AMOUNT
Neroli	2 drops
Orange	3 drops
Ylang ylang	3 drops
Cinnamon decoction	50 ml
Ginger decoction	50 ml

Rhapsody In Vanilla

OIL/BASE	AMOUNT
Black pepper	3 drops
Ylang ylang	3 drops
Rosewater	50 ml
Vanilla decoction	50 ml

Citrus Song

OIL/BASE	AMOUNT
Lime	3 drops
Petitgrain	3 drops
Orange flower water	50 ml
Vanilla decoction	50 ml

Exotic Nectar

OIL/BASE	AMOUNT
Rose	3 drops
Ylang ylang	4 drops
Vanilla decoction	100 ml

Any of the above combinations can be made with 1 teaspoon of natural vanilla extract to every 50 ml of water as a substitute for vanilla decoction.

Scented Candles

Almost all the scented candles available are perfumed with synthetic oils. From my own experience, these candles are far more likely to trigger an allergic reaction, such as wheezing or sneezing, than are candles perfumed with natural essences. Although it is possible to buy candle-making kits and to make your own essential oil candles, it is much simpler to add essential oils to the molten wax of a ready-made candle.

Try to obtain a very fat candle which will produce a good-sized pool of molten wax around the wick, thus enabling the oil to vaporize slowly. First light the candle. Wait for the wax to melt, then blow it out and immediately add a few drops of essential oil around the wick before relighting. Essential oil is highly flammable, so if you attempt to add this while the candle is still burning, it will flare up, immediately burning off the essential oil, leaving a puff of black smoke in its wake. It is also important to keep the wick of the candle trimmed very short, otherwise the flame will be too big and again, the oil will be burned too quickly, resulting in a very short-lived aromatic vapour.

As you will discover, a single candle can be used for any number of aromas. As soon as one essence (or a simple blend) has vaporized, a different one can be added if desired.

If you can obtain a pure beeswax candle, this will impart its own delicate honey scent to the surrounding air. However, beeswax candles burn down much faster than ordinary paraffin wax candles, and they are much more expensive to buy. Nevertheless, they are worth considering if you love the fragrance.

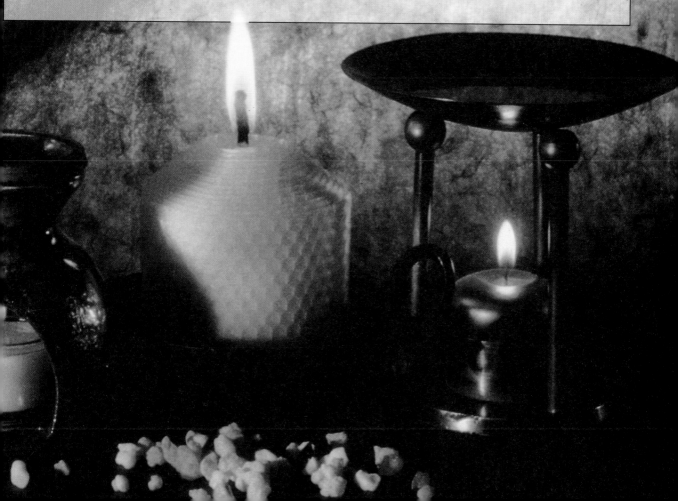

Objects of Love

You may also wish to place in a prominent position a beautiful semi-precious stone such as a piece of unpolished rose quartz, amethyst or rock crystal; or perhaps an inspiring painting, suggestive sculpture, or some other attractive art object.

If you are inspired by magical symbolism, you could choose art objects or pictures which are also representative of the god and goddess within. In India, these archetypal male and female principles are recognized in the Hindu god Shiva and his consort, the goddess Shakti – and in the lingam and the yoni. Although these last two words can also be translated as 'penis' and 'vulva', in Indian culture the meanings are much more sacred. The great lingam of Shiva is associated with the seed of creation, and the yoni of Shakti with the great womb of creation.

Here then is a partial list of suggestive objects and symbols, a few of which you may decide to use in your magical space, any of which can be used to focus your attention away from the cares of the mundane world – at least for the time set aside for yourselves. It was the

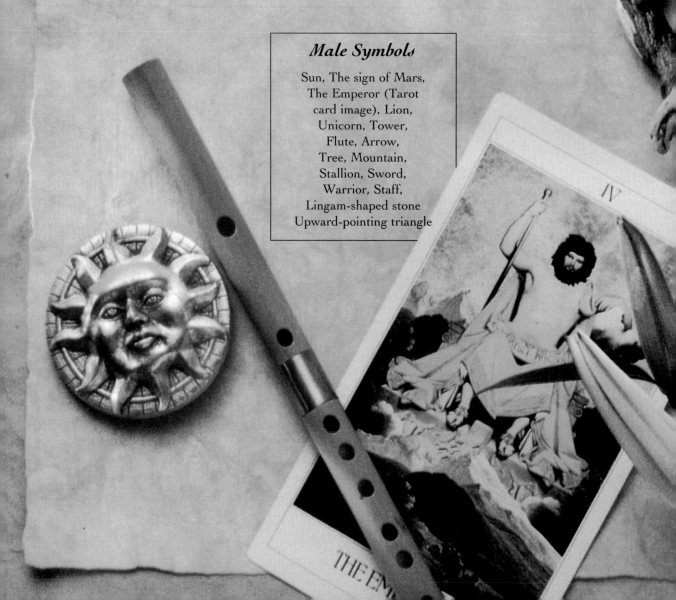

Male Symbols

Sun, The sign of Mars,
The Emperor (Tarot
card image), Lion,
Unicorn, Tower,
Flute, Arrow,
Tree, Mountain,
Stallion, Sword,
Warrior, Staff,
Lingam-shaped stone
Upward-pointing triangle

psychologist Carl Jung who proposed the reality of the psychic life, that the 'active imagination' was a path towards self-knowledge or enlightenment. He suggested that all human consciousness is linked together, that the consciousness of each person is like a small pond which trickles into the ocean of a shared 'collective unconscious'. The contents of this collective unconscious contains the archetypes. These are cross-cultural imprints, images and ideas that are intrinsic to the human psyche. These symbols based on opposites, male and female, appear in myth, fairy tales, and in world religions.

To concentrate on an archetypal object of love enables you to access the Great Lover within. The power of thought built around these symbols over thousands of years carries a psychic charge which can be harnessed to enrich your love life in very real and profound ways.

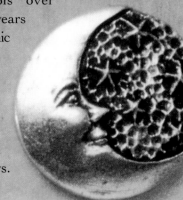

Female Symbols

Moon, The sign of Venus,
The Empress (Tarot
card image), Cup,
Star, Lotus, Hour-glass,
Sea shell, Dove,
Lily, Rose, Lute,
Yoni-shaped stone
Corn dolly, Cave,
Pearl, Boat,
Downward pointing triangle

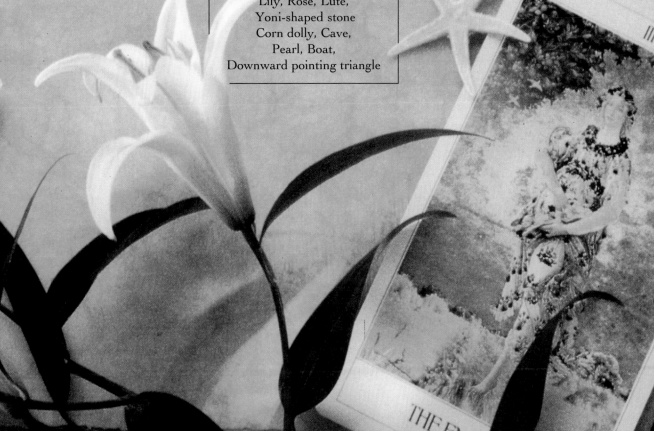

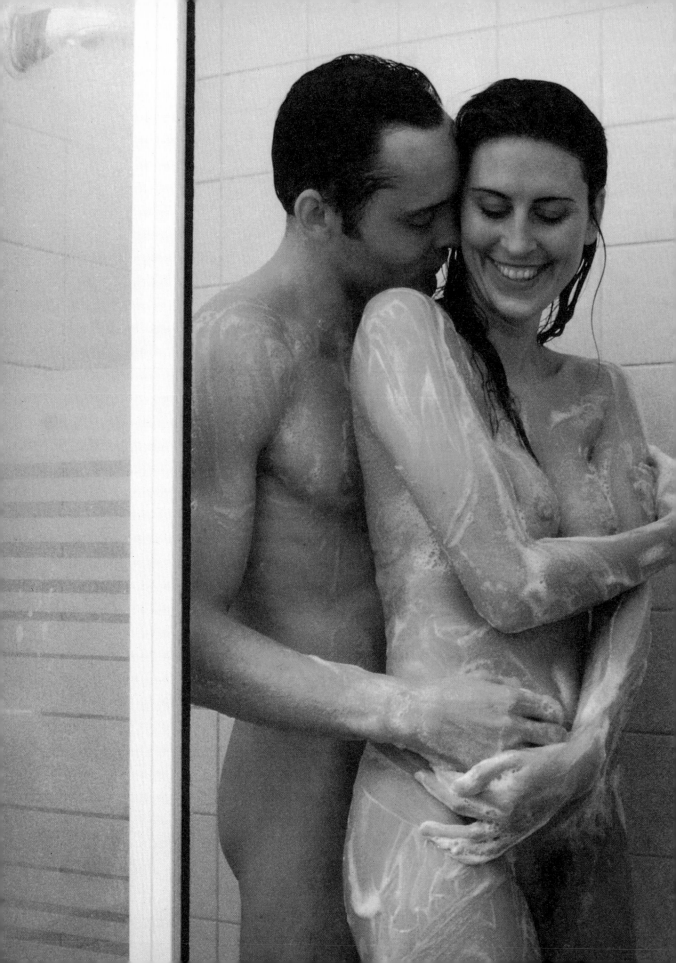

CHAPTER 6

Awakening the Senses

There is always a danger that we stick to what is familiar and don't bother to go outside the usual pattern of our lives. We would miss a great deal if we did. Out there are perfumes, tastes, sensations waiting for us to explore and experience.

Marjorie Smedley

Sensory Awakening Game

Having created your magical space, it is now time to have some fun! It is not expected that you should carry out everything in this chapter. The idea is that you pick and choose whatever takes your fancy. Most of the activities can be used as a prelude to love-making and/or erotic massage, or they can be enjoyed for their own sake. However, the exercises suggested in the last section (*see On Becoming Your Own Lover, page 95*) are more serious and are offered as a means to self-healing rather than sensual awakening. Nevertheless, they will enhance your enjoyment of lovemaking indirectly by helping to heighten your responses in general.

Any game or exercise you may choose will encourage you to be natural and childlike, to throw off the shackles of being 'grown up', at least for an hour or two. The sense of freedom and spontaneity that this can engender needs to be experienced to be believed. Not only will it enhance your lovemaking, it will encourage you to share and explore increasingly subtle levels of empathy. Indeed, true love is a feeling that there is no real distance between partners. Yet there is also the realization that both part-ners are individuals in their own right. Neither partner has power over the other. Without this seemingly paradoxical sense of intimacy and

freedom, sex can never be totally fulfilling. There will always be a yearning for more. As Margo Annand puts it: '... in reality it is not sex that opens the door to intimacy, but intimacy that opens the door to good lovemaking'.

As with erotic massage, the main purpose of the sensory awakening game that you are about to learn, is to enable you to become acquainted in a leisurely fashion with your sensual feelings – feelings that will heighten your experience of all life's pleasures, not just the experience of lovemaking. For instance: walking in the countryside and experiencing the caress of the sun on your skin; contemplat-ing the beauty of your favourite animal; listening to the voices of children happily playing; wandering by the seashore with the wind in your hair and the saltspray on your skin; and tasting the first strawberries of summer.

Moreover, when orgasm is no longer the ultimate goal, those who suffer from 'performance pressure' will experience new-found freedom. For example, if one partner is per-ceived as being too demanding sexu-ally, the other may withdraw from sex altogether, thus causing a rift in the rela-tionship. However, by learning to have

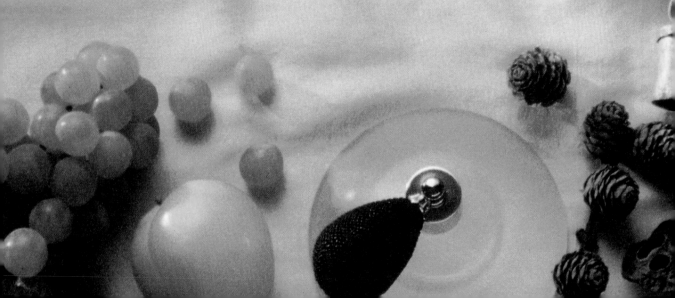

non-sexual fun together, which includes touching and being touched regularly, a great deal of tension is released. The 'demanding' partner will relax enough to passively enjoy the sensations for their own sake; and the 'unresponsive', partner, finding themselves in a non-threatening environment, will become awakened to pleasure, and most likely to their own sexual needs. And what is more, each will take delight in the other's joy – the secret of a deep and lasting relationship. In this game, both you and your partner take it in turns to introduce the other to a cornucopia of surprising and tantalizing sensory experiences. The receptive partner should be either lightly blindfolded with a silk scarf or close their eyes to enable them to focus on each sensation as it is presented. The active partner then proceeds to seduce the senses of the other with different scents, tastes, textures and sounds. When the receptive partner opens his or her eyes, the sense of sight is enhanced as a result of temporary deprivation. Rather than playing both the active and the receptive roles on the same occasion, you may prefer to play the game on two different days, perhaps taking the active role on the first day, and being receptive the second time around.

Preparation

You can create your magical space together if you wish. However, if you intend to play the sensory awakening game on two different days, you may prefer to prepare the room yourself, making this part of the treat for your lover's eyes. But even if your lover helps you to prepare the sensuous space, it is essential that they do not catch sight of anything else connected with the game. The element of surprise is vital.

As you will be awakening the sense of taste, for obvious reasons it is best not to play this game immediately after a meal. It is also important for the receptive partner to be seated comfortably because the game may go on for some time. So ensure that there is a comfortable chair for your partner to sit on, or a cushion on the floor. If you choose a cushion, it would be best to place this near a wall, which can be used to support your lover's back.

You will also need to choose music that you both find sensual and romantic. As you will be employing other sounds too, it is important to keep the volume down very low, and to regard it as background sound. Similarly, you can vaporize your lover's favourite essences, but keep the fragrance subtle, for you will also be introducing other aromas.

The only hard and fast rule of the game is to allow at least half a minute of silence before presenting a different experience, and at least one minute before moving on to a different sense. Your lover needs the chance to savour each sensation. Moreover, the anticipation of waiting for each new aroma, sound, texture or taste is the essence of the game.

Smell

As well as the oils you intend to use in the vaporizer, you will also need a few close-up aromas to be sniffed directly from the bottle or from a tissue or handkerchief. Choose essential oils you know your lover enjoys. If peppermint is a favourite, this is a good essence with which to begin because it has a piercing, awakening aroma. Other powerful essences include clove, black pepper, basil and eucalyptus. However, do not allow the oil itself to touch your lover's nostrils; undiluted essential oils can irritate the skin. It is also advisable to offer your lover no more than three or four scents. The sense of smell begins to 'fatigue' very quickly. Allow at least half a minute between each fragrance to give your lover's nose a chance to adjust.

You may also wish to include other aromas such as freshly ground coffee, Earl Grey tea, various herbs and spices, or a fragrant plant.

Hearing

For some interesting sounds, you could perhaps blow a few notes on a bamboo flute, shake a tiny bell, move some wind chimes, or make sweet sounds with any other instrument you can find. You could also blow gently across the top of a wine or milk bottle which makes a hauntingly beautiful sound like the wind blowing across moorland.

You can also use your voice, whispering sweet-nothings in your lover's ear; or perhaps read a verse or two of a sensual love poem, or an extract from an emotionally charged novel, or simply sing to your lover

Touch

For sensual touching you could include a piece of driftwood, a pine cone, coconut, smooth pebble, piece of quartz, some velvet fabric, a silk scarf, sheet of parchment-like paper, flower petals, peacock feather, a bowl of sand or anything else you can think of. As well as putting items in your lover's hand, you might also brush soft textures against their face or body, including your own hair if it is long enough. Or you could spray the surrounding air (a short distance away from your partner) with some warm, aromatic water (use a perfume atomizer or plant spray), allowing a fine mist to refresh your lover's skin.

Taste

To awaken the sense of taste, you could seduce your partner with pieces of fruit such as peach, mango, pineapple, grapes or kiwi. Or try olives, cubes of cheese, or perhaps croutons coated in a favourite dip. Offer the ambrosial morsels on a cocktail stick. Follow this with sips of wine, mead, a favourite liqueur, spring water, sparkling fruit juice, or perhaps iced coffee. If your lover has a sweet tooth, end with a piece of dark chocolate, a mint cream, some vanilla fudge, or perhaps a taste of ice-cream.

Sight

Have your lover close their eyes before entering the room then gently guide them to the place where they are to sit. Having heightened the other four senses, when your lover opens his or her eyes they will be enchanted by the surroundings. And with you too, especially if you look as otherworldly as the magical space itself. Exactly what you should wear (if anything) can be left to your imagination.

Awakening to the Dance

Dance, especially if it is undirected and free, is one of the most beautiful ways to express feelings. As well as being a superb physical and emotional release, it encourages spontaneity and freedom from self-consciousness. Sadly though, many people, men especially, feel awkward about expressing themselves in such an uninhibited way. But if we can surrender to the spirit of expressive dance, we begin to feel at ease with the lack of external structure. It can free 'masculine' people to express the caring nurturing side of their nature, while 'feminine' people can discover a sense of power and assertiveness. Thus we develop new ways of relating to ourselves, to others and the world around us. Moreover, wild and abandoned dance is an intoxicating aphrodisiac. For the freed psychic energy, hitherto locked in muscular tension and patterned ways of thinking, can be channelled into the sexual ecstatic response. How much persuasion do you need?

Up until now you have been free to choose any form of music that appeals to you, but for free expressive dance, ironically, you will need a few guidelines. The purpose of this game is to encourage expression of at least two sides of your nature – the flowing aquatic and the earthy primitive. When the body is comfortable in each, the natural flow of life can be experienced without resistance – a truly heady experience. For the flowing dance you will need music without a clear rhythmical beat – maybe a piece of slow classical or New Age music. You might find it helps to close your eyes. Simply move with the sounds, being aware of your partner. When this finishes, immediately put on some fast music with a strong rhythmic pulse of at least 90 beats a minute and move ecstatically!

The Far Pavilion

Escape from the hurly burly of city life and head for the wilds. For most lovers, a change of scene, especially close to nature, is a source of heightened erotic pleasure; you could camp on the edge of a forest, or find an isolated holiday cottage or log cabin where you can indulge your wildest fantasies, and commune with the spirits of nature. Take any of the following sensual room sprays with you to add to a perfume atomizer or plant-mister, and spray your hideaway cottage or even the inside of your tent. Add up to 20 drops of essential oil to 100 ml of water. Add the same quantity of essential oil to a 100 ml bottle of water, then use in a night-light vaporizer, for a longer-lasting, more pervasive aroma.

Sensual Room Sprays							
Use any of the blends below mixed with 100 ml of water in a perfume atomizer or a plant mister.							
Undine (water-spirit)		**Sylph** (air-spirit)		**Dryad** (tree-spirit)		**Salamander** (fire-spirit)	
OIL	DROPS	OIL	DROPS	OIL	DROPS	OIL	DROPS
Clary sage	5	Lavender	10	Cedarwood	5	Bergamot	6
Geranium	5	Lemon	5	Juniper	10	Clove	3
Lavender	10	Petitgrain	5	Patchouli	5	Lavender	6

Water Play

The possibilities for sensuous and fragrant pleasure in the bath or shower are limitless, and can be a prelude to an erotic massage and lovemaking, or pleasurable in their own right. Have fun in the shower, or take an aromatic bath with your lover. Luxuriate in the heady scents, combined with the silky warmth of the water against your skin and that of your lover. Wash each other's hair or give one another a sensual scalp massage using one of the hair tonic blends (*see Chapter 4*). A neck massage given or received in the bath can be a deeply relaxing experience as well as an incredibly erotic one. Use one of the essential oil combinations specially blended for your particular skin type (*see Chapter 4*). You can further

enhance the setting if you bathe by candlelight – use scented candles to surround yourself with sensual, heady fragrance.

It can also be deliciously erotic to share a ripe juicy peach or luscious strawberries in the bath. Just let the juices flow everywhere – it will all come out in the wash.

Afterwards, dry each other with scented towels. The simplest way to perfume towels is to spray them with a perfume atomizer or mister. Add up to 5 drops of essential oil to 30 ml of water, place in your atomizer, shake well, then spray a fine mist over the towels. Allow them to dry in a warm airing cupboard or on a heated towel rail before using them. The warmth will bring out the aroma. (*Continued on page 94*)

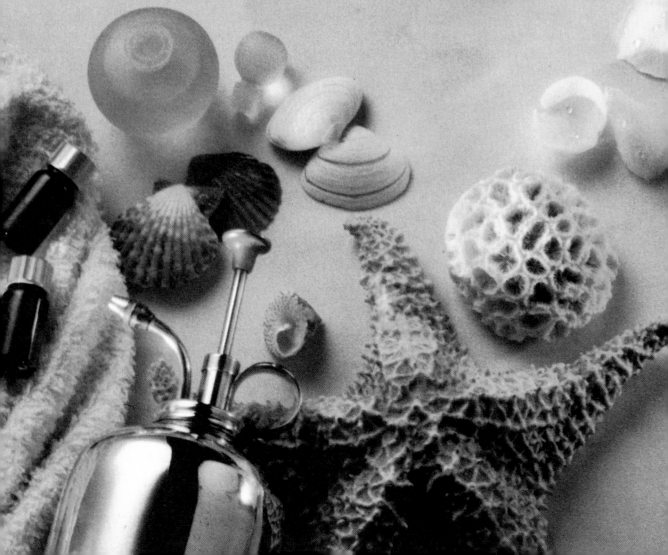

CHAPTER 7

Erotic Massage with Essential Oils

My lover put his hand to the doorhole
and my body thrilled and moved
I rose up to my beloved
my hands dripped with myrrh
fingers of sweet myrrh grasped the handle

Max Lake (after *The Song of Songs*)

The Art of Sensual Massage

You have created your magical space, perhaps bathed or showered and are now ready to explore the delights of aromatic massage. The sequence you are about to learn is a modified form of therapeutic massage – eroticized through the power of intent and the spirit of playfulness. But contrary to what the ancient erotic texts proclaim, no matter how skilled you may become in the art of sensual massage, it will never be a 'turn-on' for another person if there is no real chemistry between you, and if there is no love or tenderness in your touch.

However, for a couple going through a bad patch, loving touch (not necessarily erotic massage) can impart that vital element of mutual trust and relaxation which may have fallen by the wayside – or perhaps never quite developed in the first place. Indeed, too many people equate cuddling, touching and massage as a prelude to sexual intercourse rather than as a means of fulfilling a need for sensual contact, independent of an ultimate goal. However, for the couple who already have a wonderful relationship, massage will enhance and intensify the loving bond in a way that words cannot possibly describe.

Preparing the Room

The room in which you intend to exchange massage should be very warm. Even though the temperature may be warm enough for normal purposes, it is surprisingly easy to become chilled when unclothed and lying still for any length of time, especially with oil on your skin. So unless it is a sweleringly hot day (or night) do take this into account. The aim of erotic massage is to make your lover quiver with pleasure rather than shiver with cold!

Work in natural daylight or under a soft lamp or candlelight. If you live in a noisy area, you may wish to camouflage any background disturbance by playing a tape of gentle music. It is vital to keep the volume down very low – your lover's senses will be especially acute. And do not forget to unplug the phone.

The Massage Surface

Although a professional massage therapist would use a purpose-made massage couch, this is hardly conducive to eroticism. So it is best to work at floor level, on a futon or on a bed with a firm mattress. Should you decide to give massage on the floor, a sleeping-bag, strip of foam rubber, thick blankets, a soft rug or a folded double-sized duvet will provide the necessary padding under your partner. Cover this with a sheet or a couple of fluffy bath towels. You may also need a second sheet or bath towel to cover areas of the body you are not working on, thus preventing your lover from becoming chilled. This may not be necessary if the room is extremely warm, or if your lover is hot-blooded! Should you decided to massage your lover on the bed, you may still wish to place a towel under their body to protect the sheets from oil stains.

When giving massage, kneel beside your partner: preferably on a carpeted floor to cushion your knees, or on the bed. However, do not attempt to give massage while standing and bending at the waist. Apart from impeding the all-important flow of the massage, it puts an enormous strain on the lower back.

The Massage Oil

Essential oils are never used neat for massage; they must be first diluted in a good quality vegetable oil base. The basic instructions for preparing massage oils are to be found in Chapter 4. Although personal preference is vital when choosing oils for erotic massage, in the following box are a few tried and tested sensual blends just to inspire you. But do not

Sensual Massage Blends

Choose one of the blends suggested below, or mix one of your own creations.
You may prefer to use infused oil of vanilla as a base for your essential oil blends (*see page 147*).
Quantities of essential oils are given in drops for 25 ml of base oil.

Arabian Nights

OILS	DROPS
Coriander	3
Frankincense	3
Lime	2
Rose	2

Tonight Josephine

OILS	DROPS
Bergamot	2
Jasmine	4
Lavender	2
Petitgrain	2

Titania

OILS	DROPS
Bergamot	3
Lavender	2
Neroli	3
Vetiver	1

Velvet Seduction

OILS	DROPS
Rose	2
Sandalwood	5
Ylang Ylang	2

Eros

OILS	DROPS
Coriander	3
Ginger	1
Sandalwood	6

Sultry Nights and Roses

OILS	DROPS
Geranium	3
Patchouli	2
Rose	3

forget to mix a lower concentration of essences for facial massage, taking into account your lover's skin type (*see the Skin-care Chart on page 68*) and his or her preferences.

Conscious Breathing

Before giving or receiving massage, the following breathing exercise will help you to connect with your physical sensations, thus enhancing your capacity to be sensual. Conscious breathing also switches attention from any distracting thoughts or worries, and so enables you to focus fully on the pleasure of massage – and also on lovemaking. Do the exercise together with your lover.

Wear loose fitting clothing (or nothing at all) so as not to constrict your breathing. Put on some soft music that you know will last for no longer than ten minutes (perhaps towards the end of a longer composition). This is the length of time you will need for the exercise to be of any benefit.

1 Sit in your sensuous space, opposite one another, cross-legged on the floor if you can – or on a chair if you are more comfortable this way. Your posture should be upright without slouching to facilitate even, steady breathing.

2 Close your eyes and take some deep breaths. Become aware of your abdomen as it rises and falls with each breath. Clear your mind and focus only on your breathing.

3 Breathe in through your nose, but do not force it; allow yourself to breathe slowly but naturally. With each out-breath count silently to yourself. Breathe in and out and count 'one'; in and out again and count 'two' and so on up to ten. Count only on the out-breath. Once you reach ten, go back to one again. If you lose count or thoughts come flooding into your mind, gently push them aside and start again with one.

4 When the music has stopped, very slowly bring back your consciousness into the present surroundings. Open your eyes, slowly stretch out your body and begin the massage when you are ready.

The Gesture of Massage

The simple full-body sequence you are about to learn allows plenty of scope for relying on your own natural inclination. It is based on four massage movements: stroking (using the whole of the hand), kneading (rhythmic squeezing), friction (using the ball of the thumbs) and feathering (light fingertip stroking).

These movements in themselves are not necessarily erotic and can be used simply to relax your lover after a harrowing day. But add very light scratching, licking, hot breath on the skin, and other diversions – fired with an overwhelming desire for your lover – then before you know it, you are courting Eros!

A few books on sensual massage advocate stimulation of certain 'trigger points' that relate specifically to healthy sexual function. For instance, firm thumb pressure at a point five centimetres (two inches) above the crease of the buttocks is said to heighten sexual response in women, whereas thumb pressure to the point halfway between the pubic bone and navel is said to increase sexual vigour in men. Unless you are artful, your lover may perceive this action as a form of clinical prodding, a demand for them to 'turn on' – or else! Far better to give a slow, rhythmic massage which also includes attention to the erogenous zones: the lower abdomen, insides of the thighs, backs of knees, buttocks, lower back, breasts, ears, lips, back of neck, palms, insides of elbows, armpits, soles of the feet and in between the toes and the fingers.

But do try to avoid direct touching of the genitals. The purpose of erotic massage is to caress and tease your lover, to slowly but surely build up a sexual charge from the top of the head to the tips of the toes – a powerful preliminary to ecstatic sexual release.

You will find that with practice you will quickly gain confidence, even though your first movements may at first seem uncertain. Once you are able to relax into the movements, your touch will feel good no matter how basic the strokes. By trying out the massage movements on each other, you will begin to develop a sense of how massage should feel. Generally speaking, what feels good to you should also feel good to your lover. Yet it has to be acknowledged that there may be some truth in the traditionally-held idea that women are more responsive to lingering, gentle stimulation, while men prefer firmer handling. But you must discover for yourself what you and your lover find erotic.

Timing

If you were to miss out the obviously sexy parts of the sequence – lingering fingertip brushing of the thighs and breasts, and such like – and were to concentrate on firm kneading of the neck, shoulders, back and legs, you could spend about an hour relaxing your lover. But they may be too sleepy to return the compliment, at least until the next day. Erotic massage, on the other hand, is designed to arouse rather than to sedate – and this can occur quite quickly. Nevertheless, do try to give each other at least fifteen minutes (preferably half an hour) of exquisite teasing before moving on to other things.

A Few Tips

Never give massage (erotic or otherwise) while feeling anxious, angry, depressed or irritable. Your partner will pick up your feelings and will begin to feel equally distressed. Never apply the massage oil directly on to your partner's body; instead, pour a small amount into the palm of your hand, to warm the oil, then rub your hands together to ensure that they have enough oil to make massage possible. Ask your lover to remove all jewellery and contact lenses before you start your massage.

When applying the oil in long smooth strokes, try to keep the whole of your hands in contact with your lover's body, moulding its contours just as if you were sculpting clay.

When you need to apply more oil, try not to break contact with your lover's body. Keep one hand on their back, for instance, or arm, foot or head. Ideally, the whole massage should feel like a continuous flowing movement. To break contact mid-flow will feel most disconcerting to your partner. However, it is fine to break contact once you have reached a natural break in the sequence, i.e. when you have finished working on the back of the body and you wish your lover to turn over.

Add interest by varying the pressure from very light to very strong. It should be lighter over bony areas, such as the shins and knees, but quite firm over large muscles such as those either side of the spine and the buttocks. But never apply pressure to the spine itself. Slow movements are calming; fast movements are bracing; very slow and deliberate movements are sensual.

Work with your whole body, not just your hands and arms. For instance, when you are kneading, move gently from side to side in time with your hands. Allow your natural rhythm to come to the fore.

If you can remember to synchronize your breathing with the movement of your hands, your touch will be perceived as flowing, relaxed and confident. For instance, when sliding over the legs or the back, exhale slowly as you lean into the stroke; inhale as you release the pressure on the return stroke. Try not to hold your breath while doing the sliding strokes (a common mistake) as this creates tension in the hands. The tension will then be conveyed to your lover.

Remember that sensitivity combined with the sheer pleasure of giving massage, no matter how basic, far outweighs a full routine of complicated strokes if they are carried out in a mechanical manner.

When Not To Massage

Massage is contra-indicated in the following conditions: fever, inflammation (of skin or joints), thrombosis, phlebitis, varicose veins, skin ulcers, rashes or eruptions, swellings, bruises, sprains, torn muscles and ligaments, broken bones and burns – in short, if it hurts, abandon the movement and move on to another area of the body.

Although it is tempting to try and follow the massage stokes with the book propped up in front of you, your lover will experience this as a series of disconnected rubs rather than a sensual massage. It is far better to study the pictures and instructions first, maybe practising the main strokes on your own legs. Once you have developed a feel for the strokes, try them out on your partner. It is best to begin with just one area of the body at a time, rather than trying to complete a full-body massage, until you have built up your confidence. A good place to start learning is on the back, where you have a large area to stroke. If you are in any doubt about what to do next just continue stroking; as long as your movements are confident and rhythmic, your touch will feel good.

Attunement

Before oiling your hands, move to the right of your lover and place your left hand gently on the crown of his or her head. Place your right hand on the base of the spine. Breathe slowly and deeply, allowing yourself to relax. Keep your hands in place for about half a minute. This has a calming effect on both of you, and at the same time, encourages your lover to focus on your touch.

Back and Buttocks

Since most massage strokes can be used on the back, this is a good place to begin learning the art of sensual massage. Ask your lover to lie on his or her front, head to one side, arms relaxed at the sides.

1 MAIN PICTURE *Oil your hands with the blend, then position yourself at your lover's head. Gently place your warm hands horizontally on either side of the spine on the topmost part of the back, fingers pointing towards spine. Using a sliding stroke, move your hands down the length of the back, and over the buttocks.*

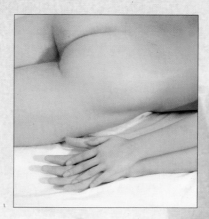

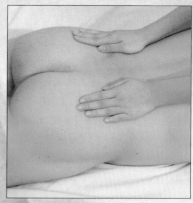

3 *When you reach the hands, slide your fingers in between your lover's fingers, then lightly glide your fingertips up the inside of the arms. When you reach the shoulders, pivot your hands back to the starting position. Repeat several times.*

4 *Continue by sliding your hands down to the buttocks and, again using sliding strokes, move your hands in wide circles, letting the circles overlap as your hands move up and over the shoulders forming a continuous spiral pattern. Repeat several times.*

2 *Glide hands out over the hips and slowly pull them up the sides of the body and into the armpits. Fan your hands out over your lover's shoulders, then lightly glide them down the outer edge of the arms.*

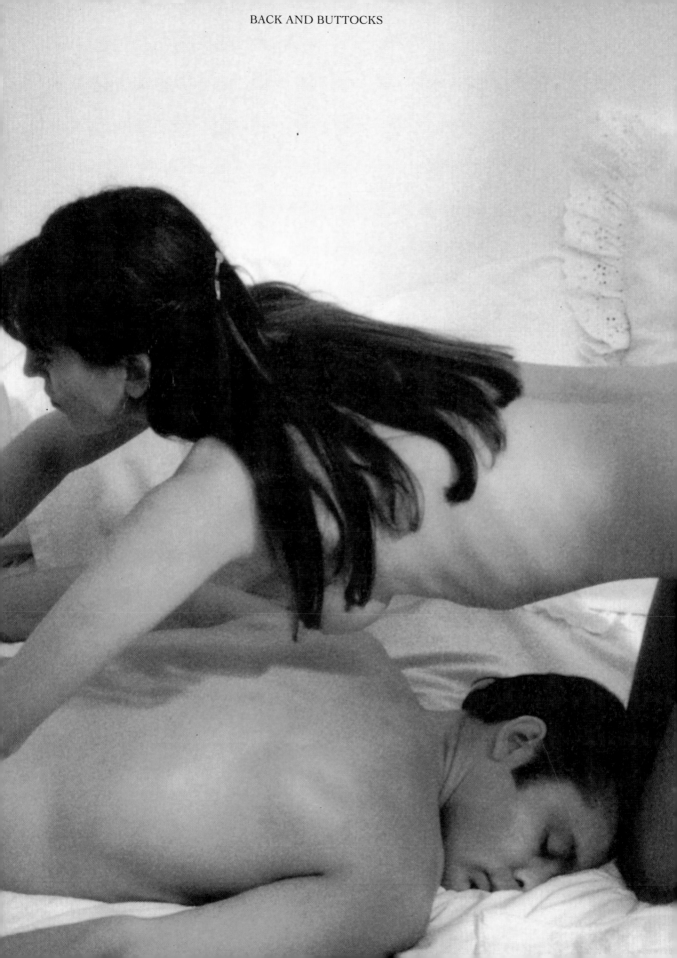

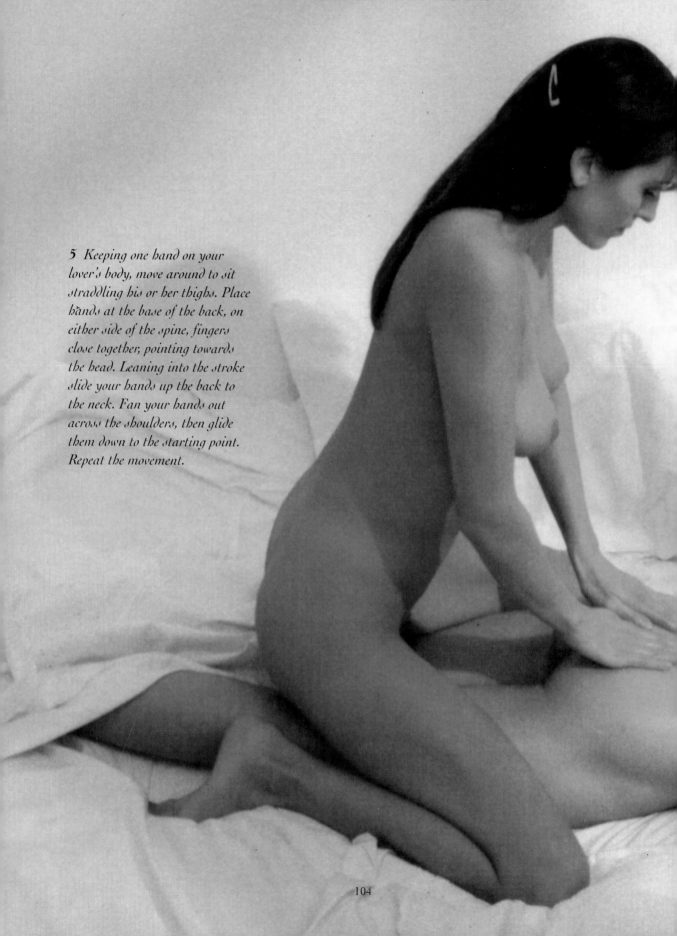

5 *Keeping one hand on your lover's body, move around to sit straddling his or her thighs. Place hands at the base of the back, on either side of the spine, fingers close together, pointing towards the head. Leaning into the stroke slide your hands up the back to the neck. Fan your hands out across the shoulders, then glide them down to the starting point. Repeat the movement.*

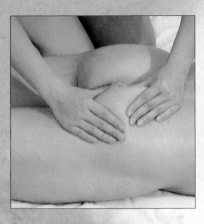
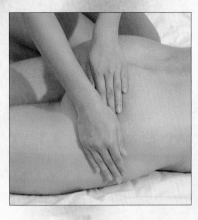

6 *Move to one side of your lover's body. Starting at the buttocks and moving up the side of the body, knead the fleshy or muscular parts by alternately squeezing and releasing handfuls of flesh in a broad circular motion. This relaxes tense muscles by draining away waste products.*

7 *Still in the same position, place your hands on one buttock. Gently pull each hand alternately straight up, each time overlapping the place where the last hand was. Place hands on opposite buttock and work your way slowly up to the armpit and back down again. Repeat on the other side.*

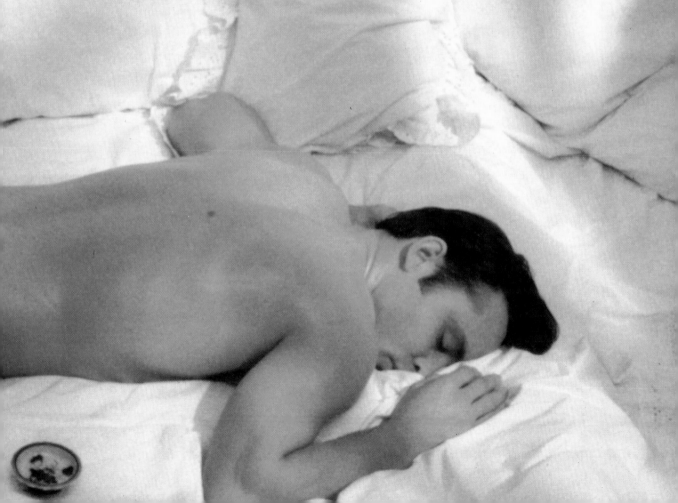

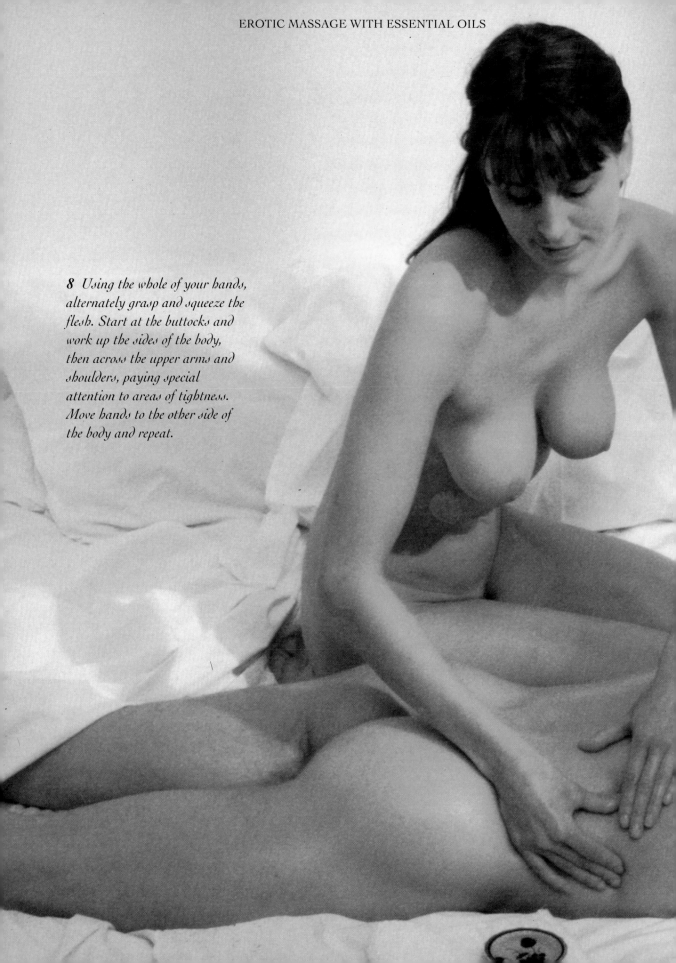

8 *Using the whole of your hands, alternately grasp and squeeze the flesh. Start at the buttocks and work up the sides of the body, then across the upper arms and shoulders, paying special attention to areas of tightness. Move hands to the other side of the body and repeat.*

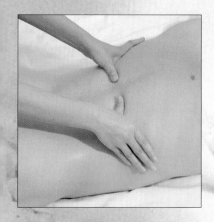 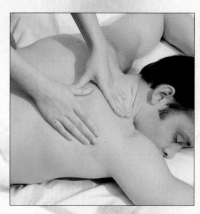 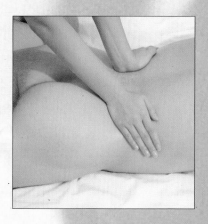

9 *Sit straddling your lover's thighs. Place hands on lower back, thumbs towards each other, on either side of spine. Lean into the stroke as you slide up the back to the neck, then fan your hands out across shoulders, ease the pressure and slide back down to the starting position. Repeat.*

10 *From base of spine, make small circular movements with thumbs on either side of the spine up to neck. With thumbs on upper back, continue circular movement. Do not press on spine or shoulder-blade, work on muscles just above the shoulder-blades and those lying between them and spine.*

11 *Return to sliding stroke (step 5) and repeat. Apply fairly strong pressure to lower back by circling with heels of your hands. Using thumbs as before, work on any areas of tension in buttocks and lower back. Continue with several sliding strokes up the back.*

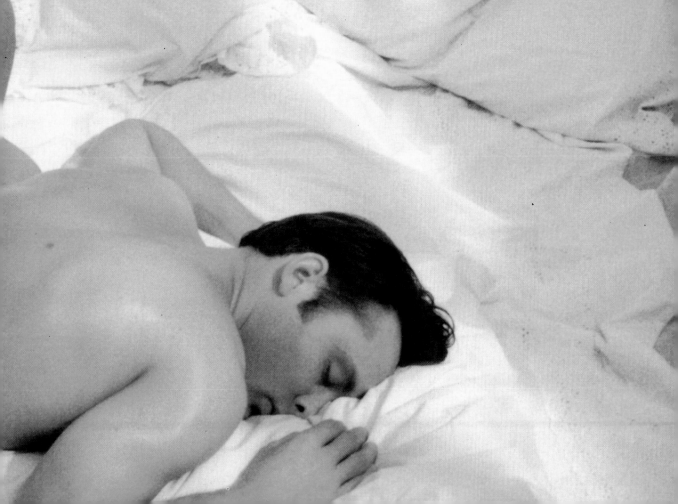

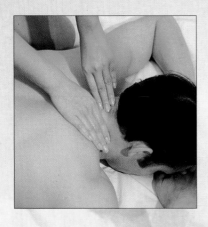

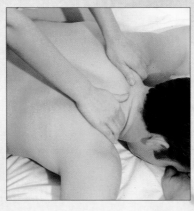

14 Ask your lover to release hands and place his or her head to one side as before. Knead both shoulders at the same time. Move into position straddling your lover's thighs. Repeat step 5 sliding your hands up the back and down the sides of the body.

12 Sit to one side of your lover. Ask your lover to rest his or her forehead on hands. Knead the neck muscles by working on shoulders and up the neck to the base of the skull.

13 Using both hands, knead the sides of the neck, up to the base of the skull. Keep the strokes fluid and the pressure fairly consistent.

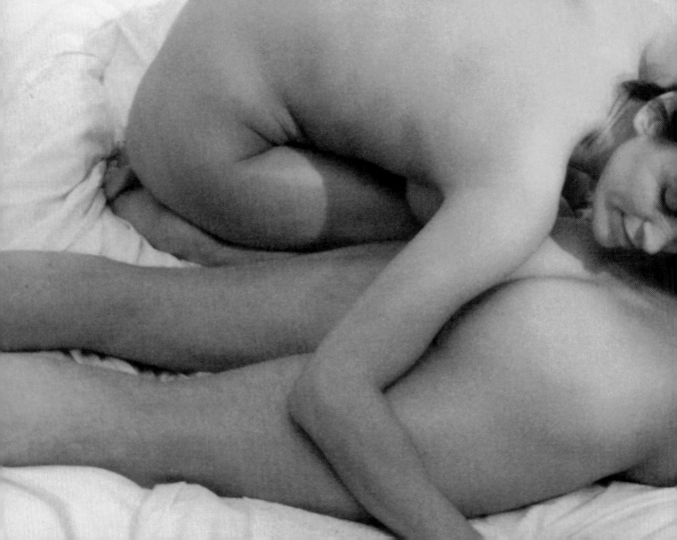

15 MAIN PICTURE *Now you can begin to have some fun. Feathering or light caressing can be done with long hair, or even with a bushy beard! So, if either you or your lover qualify, slowly caress the other's body by sweeping your hair (or beard) over it. Brush from the top of the neck and down the body to the tips of the toes before starting again. Do not forget to sweep down each arm as well. Repeat as many times as you wish .*

16 *Using delicate strokes of the hands, softly stroke the neck, then kiss and nibble the nape of the neck. Repeat the gentle strokes, then the soft kisses.*

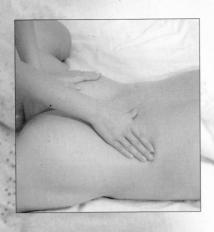

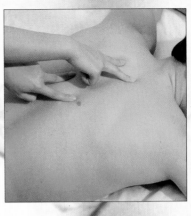

17 *Straddling your lover's thighs, place one hand on hip, while using the thumb of your other hand to snake up the spine. Start at the tail bone and trace your finger in and out of spaces between vertebrae up the spine to the base of the skull, but do not press too hard over the spine.*

18 *Then using your index and middle fingertips, press down firmly on either side of the spine with one hand overlapping the path of the other. Go all the way down to the lower end of the spine and off at the tail bone. Repeat this step several times up and down the spine.*

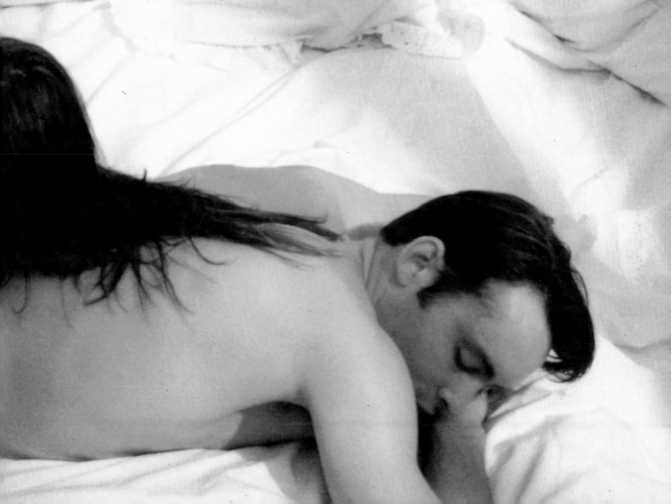

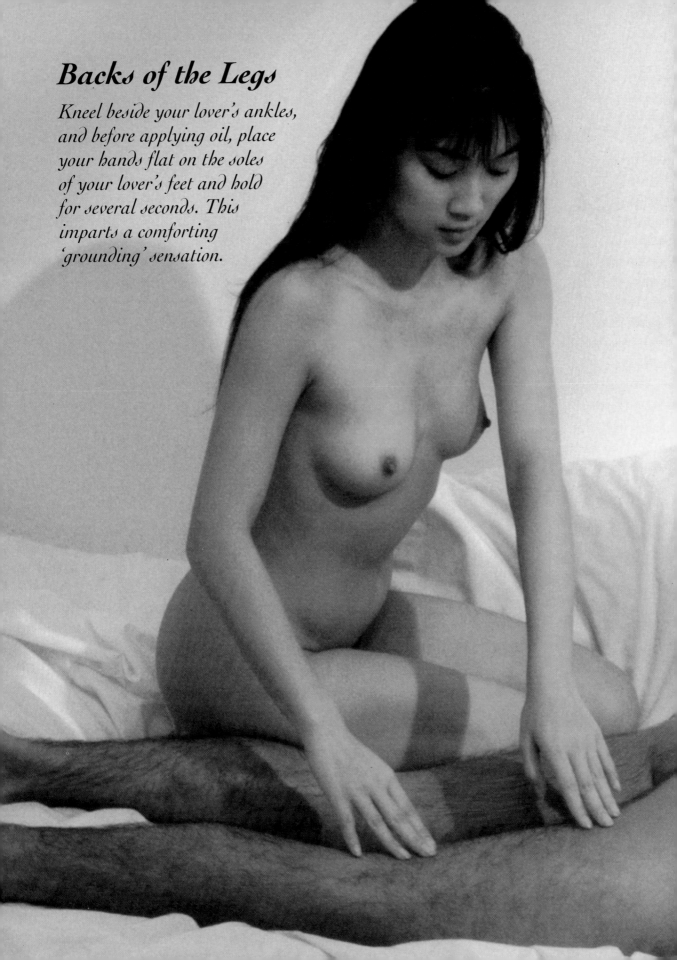

Backs of the Legs

Kneel beside your lover's ankles, and before applying oil, place your hands flat on the soles of your lover's feet and hold for several seconds. This imparts a comforting 'grounding' sensation.

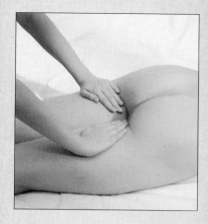 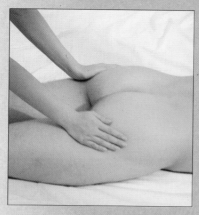 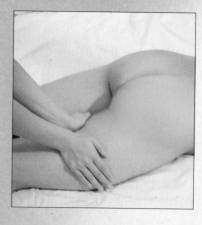

1 Oil your hands. Starting at ankles, place your right hand on your lover's right leg and left hand on left leg, hands pivoted so that fingers cup the inner sides of ankles. Leaning into the stroke, slide both hands together firmly up the legs.

2 When you reach the crease of the buttocks, slide your hands around so that the fingers point towards the head, and glide lightly down the outer side of the legs and off at the ankles. Repeat this movement several times, applying more oil if necessary.

3 Use your thumbs to apply friction to the calf muscles of one leg. Press gently, moving your thumbs away from you in short alternating strokes all the way up to the back of the knee. This is a very tender spot, so never apply pressure here.

4 When you reach the thighs, press heels of your hands into the muscles, using broad deep strokes. Knead the thigh, gently on the inner part, strongly on outer part where muscles are larger. Knead calf muscles with both hands, using rhythmical movements.

5 MAIN PICTURE Do some feather-light stroking with fingertips barely touching the skin, paying special attention to inner thighs and backs of knees. Then feather the whole body, until your lover is tingling with sexual sensitivity!

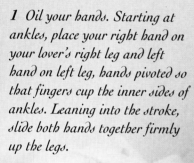
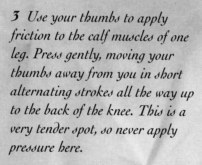

Fronts of the Legs

Ask your lover to lie on his or her back, with arms comfortably at sides and legs outstretched in a relaxed position. Take more care on the front of the body, especially with sensitive abdomen and breast/chest areas.

1 MAIN PICTURE *Oil your hands and kneel beside your partner's ankles. Starting on one leg, cup your hands over the ankle and stroke up the front of the leg, one hand overlapping the path of the other. Do not apply direct pressure to the shin bone as this can be painful. Repeat several times, applying more oil if necessary.*

2 *When you reach the top of the thigh, fan your hands out and glide them lightly down the sides. Repeat several times, then move on to work on the other leg, starting at step 1.*

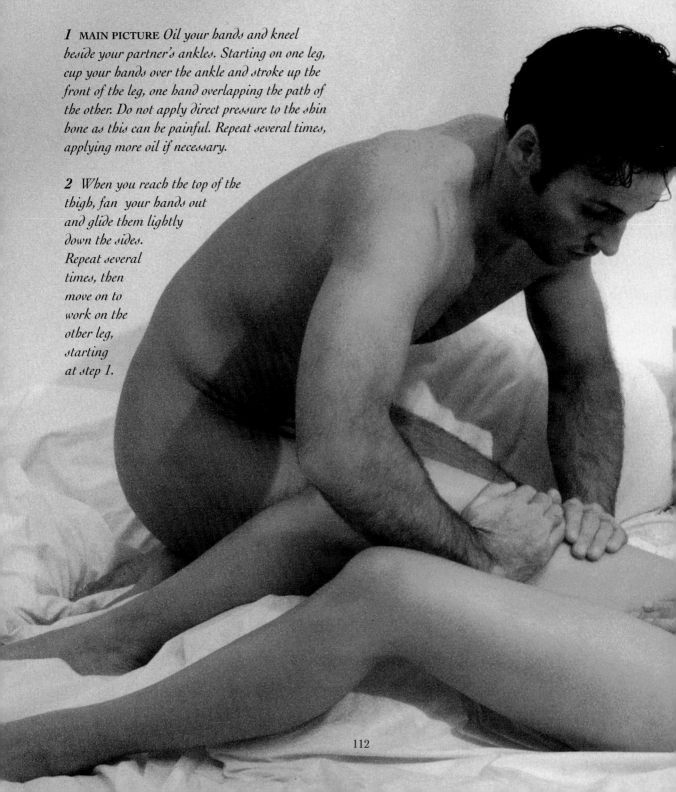

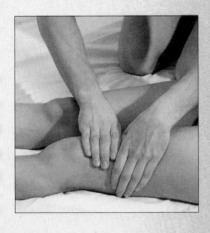
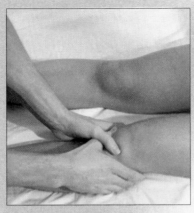
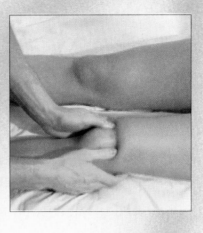

3 Return to the thigh of one leg and place your hands, fingers facing away from you, on either side of it. Now push firmly with left hand and pull back with your right. Without stopping, change the position of your hands and push-and-pull in opposite directions. Return to a stroking movement as in step 1.

4 Start with your thumbs crossed just under the knee. Stroke up sides of knee to the top, one thumb on each side, allowing your thumbs to pass at the top.

5 Now stroke each thumb down the opposite side, both thumbs completing a full circle, passing the other at the tops and bottom. Repeat. Continue with circular thumb pressures around the knee.

6 Lovingly stroke the sides and back of the knee with fingers of both hands at once. Complete the sequence by stroking the entire leg from ankle to thigh. Repeat the sequence on the other leg.

7 Do featherlight stroking with the fingertips over each leg. Teasingly brush past the genitals, but pay special attention to the inner and outer thighs and the fronts of the knees.

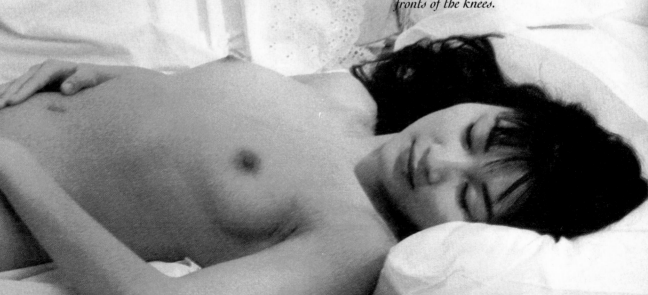

Feet

A foot massage is extremely relaxing and very pleasurable. Unless the skin is exceptionally dry, the foot requires very little oil. Place your lover's foot in your lap, or if it is easier keep the foot on the massage surface.

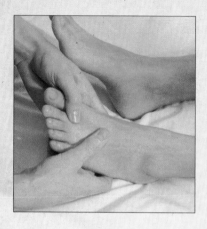 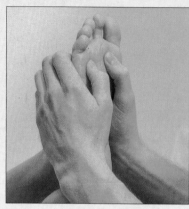 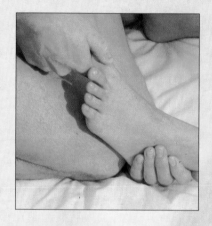

1 Begin by stroking your lover's right foot. Hold it between your hands and stroke firmly with both hands from the toes towards the body. When you reach the ankles, return your hands to the toes with a light stroke. Repeat. Then support the foot by placing your fingers underneath it with your thumbs on top at the base of the toes (above). Moving towards the ankle, make broad circles all over the top of the foot.

2 Work on the soles of the foot with the thumbs of both hands. Make small circles covering the entire sole. Pinch the outer edge of the heel, continuing all the way up the outer edge of the foot to the little toe.

3 Now work on the toes. Starting with the big toe, gently squeeze and roll each toe between your thumb and index finger; rotate each one very gently in both directions, then pull each toe gently towards you.

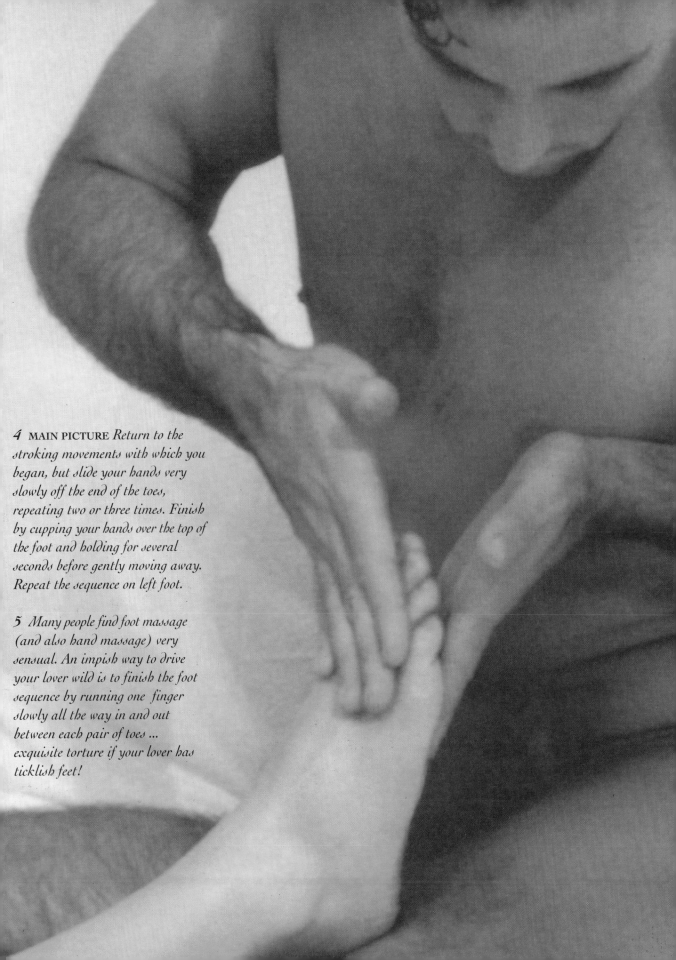

4 MAIN PICTURE *Return to the stroking movements with which you began, but slide your hands very slowly off the end of the toes, repeating two or three times. Finish by cupping your hands over the top of the foot and holding for several seconds before gently moving away. Repeat the sequence on left foot.*

5 *Many people find foot massage (and also hand massage) very sensual. An impish way to drive your lover wild is to finish the foot sequence by running one finger slowly all the way in and out between each pair of toes ... exquisite torture if your lover has ticklish feet!*

Arms and Hands

Oil your hands and position yourself beside your lover's upper thighs. Although the arms will require oil, the hands, like the feet, require very little.

1 MAIN PICTURE *Holding your lover's hand in one hand and massaging with the other, slide your hand up the arm from wrist to shoulder. When you reach the top, glide back down the outer edge of the arm and off at the wrist. Repeat.*

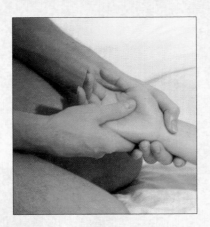

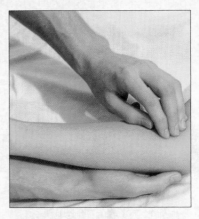

2 *Holding the wrist in one hand, circle the centre of the palm with your thumb. Extend these circular thumb pressures over the whole palm and up on to the forearm. Now, using both hands, knead the forearm, working from the wrist to the elbow, then slide your hand down to start again. Then knead the upper arm. Repeat several times.*

3 *Massage the elbow by circling with your fingers. Use plenty of oil as the skin here is usually very dry. Then massage the insides of the elbows using gentle circular strokes. Return to the sliding movement with which you began, and repeat several times. Repeat the sequence from step 1 on the other arm.*

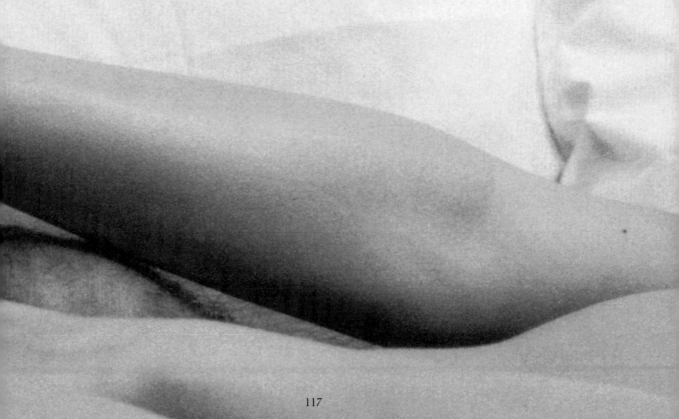

4 MAIN PICTURE *Caress your lover's hands and arms with soft lips and hot breath on the skin.*

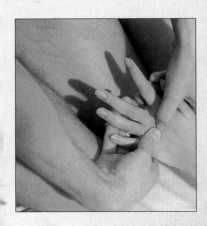
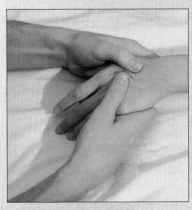
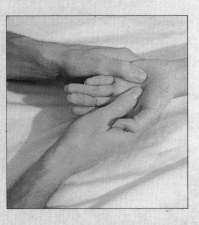

5 *With both thumbs lying horizontally over the knuckle, press down and at the same time, flex the finger towards you, giving your lover's hand a good stretch.*

6 *Massage the back of your lover's hand by rotating your thumbs in tiny circles over the back of the hand, the fingers and the wrist.*

7 *Turn the palm uppermost, paying attention to the muscular base of the thumb, circle the palm with your thumbs, then circle more gently over the inner wrist.*

8 *Hold your lover's hand, palm down in one hand and using your other to work on each finger. Paying particular attention to each joint, do circular thumb pressures along the top of each finger, from the tip to the knuckle. Squeeze the outer edge of each finger, then gently pull them, giving a little twist as you slide your hand down and off the fingertips. Repeat sequence on each finger then on the other hand.*

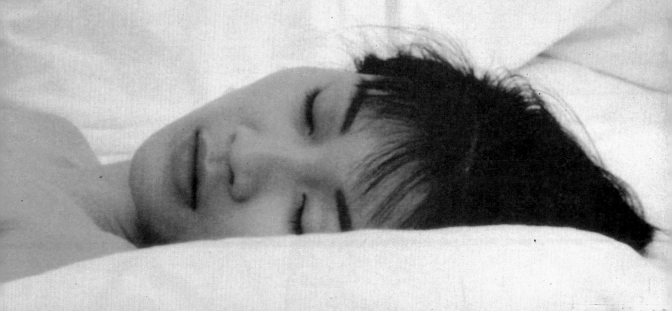

Face and Head, Neck and Shoulders

Only the lightest fingertip pressure is required for the face, and it is particularly important not to drag the delicate skin. Use firm pressure over the scalp.

1 MAIN PICTURE *Position yourself behind your lover's head. Start with your hands lying next to each other horizontally across the area just below the collar-bone, tips of the fingers touching. Slide your hands apart, moving across the top of the shoulders and up the back of the neck. Repeat.*

2 Starting from the throat and sweeping up to the chin, using the whole of your hands, slide over the face. Circle the cheeks, moving round the eyes (but not close enough for oil to seep in) and over the forehead. This will oil the skin before you begin the main part of the massage.

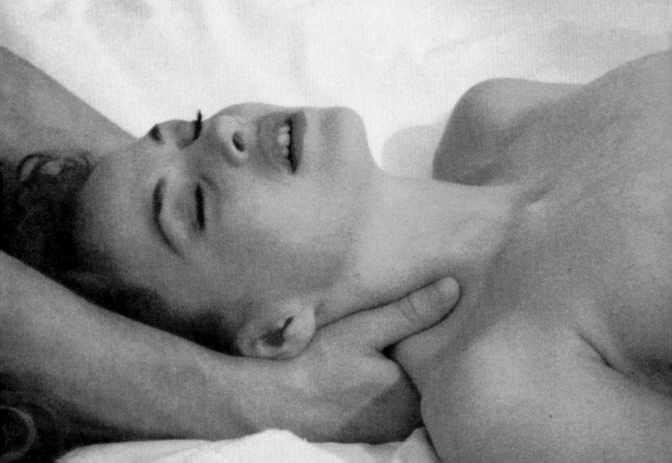

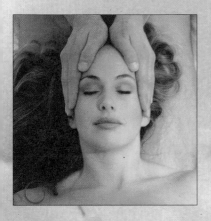
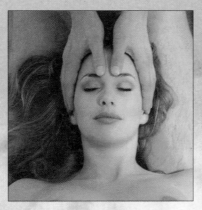
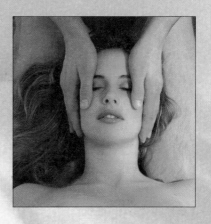

3 Place your hands on either side of your lover's head, the heels of the hands covering the forehead, the fingers extending downwards, anchoring the sides of the head. Hold them there for a few moments, then move your hands to the forehead and smoothly stroke the brow, hand over hand, up and over the hair to the crown of the head.

4 Place the ball of your thumbs at the centre of the forehead between eyebrows. Slide both thumbs apart and when you reach the temples, finish with a circular flourish before gliding off at the hairline. Return to the starting position, but this time a little higher up, continue to stroke the forehead, a strip at a time, all the way up to the hairline.

5 Place the ball of your thumbs below the inner corners of the eyes. Smooth towards the temples. Repeat a little lower down, a strip at a time, until you reach the cheek-bones. Repeat below the bone, pressing lightly. Using your middle fingers, make tiny circles down the sides of nose, at either side of the nostrils and over upper lip. Then place thumbs on chin and pull slowly along jaw-bone to ear. Repeat further up until just below the cheek-bone. Then work in tiny circles with thumbs, from the middle of chin along the jaw-bone, finishing behind the ears.

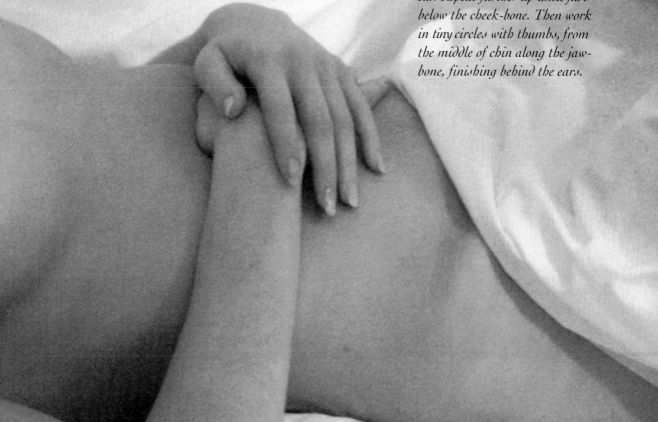

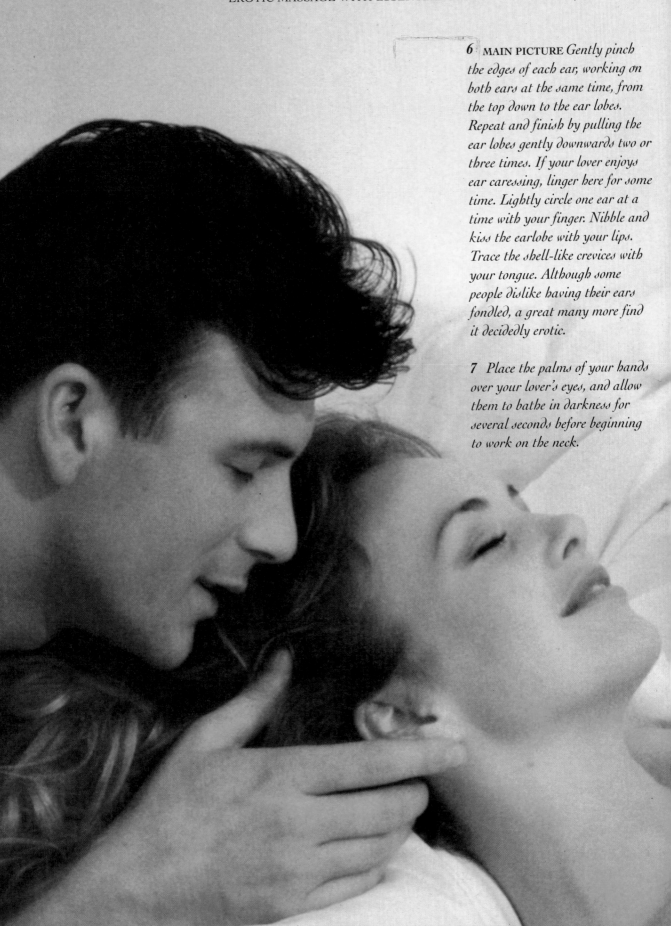

6 MAIN PICTURE *Gently pinch the edges of each ear, working on both ears at the same time, from the top down to the ear lobes. Repeat and finish by pulling the ear lobes gently downwards two or three times. If your lover enjoys ear caressing, linger here for some time. Lightly circle one ear at a time with your finger. Nibble and kiss the earlobe with your lips. Trace the shell-like crevices with your tongue. Although some people dislike having their ears fondled, a great many more find it decidedly erotic.*

7 *Place the palms of your hands over your lover's eyes, and allow them to bathe in darkness for several seconds before beginning to work on the neck.*

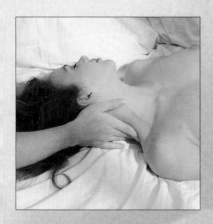
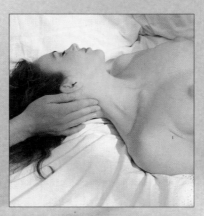
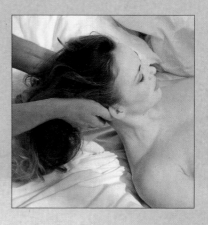

8 *Gently turn your lover's head to the left. Place your left hand on the forehead, or, if you prefer, support the head by letting it rest in your left hand. Place your right hand on your lover's right shoulder and slide your hand firmly all the way up to the neck.*

9 *When you reach the base of the skull, use all your fingers and gently circle the area several times to release any muscle tension. Return to gliding movement in step 10 and repeat before turning your lover's head to the right. Repeat 10 and 11 on the left side.*

10 *Gently move your lover's head to the middle so that the neck is straight. Give the neck a good stretch by clasping your hands together at the back of neck and lift head a few inches from massage surface; pull base of skull smoothly towards you. Still supporting the head, allow it to come back down gently. Repeat.*

11 *Next, using both hands at the back of the skull, lift your lover's head slowly forward as far as it will comfortably go before allowing it to come gently down on to the massage surface.*

12 *There is no need to oil the scalp. Simply lift your lover's head and turn it gently to the left. Press the scalp quite firmly with your fingers, moving fingers and scalp together over the skull. Repeat on the other side, then move the head back to the centre. Run your fingers through your lover's hair several times, allowing your fingers to brush the scalp gently.*

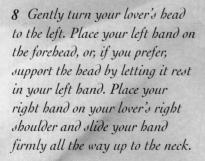
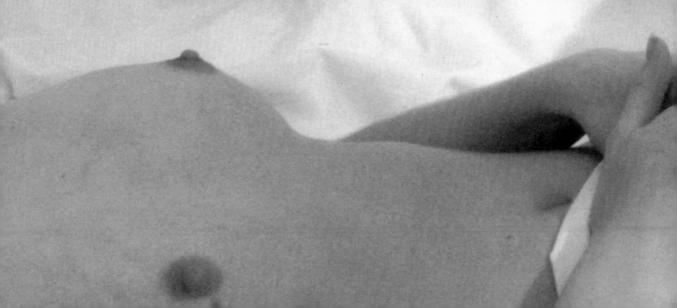

Breast and Belly

Some people are a little apprehensive about having this sensitive area massaged. If your lover is one of them, use only the lightest loving touch.

1 MAIN PICTURE *After caressing your lover's ears, glide your hands very lightly over the throat and onto the chest, fingers pointing towards the feet. Slide your hands very slowly over the breasts or chest, down towards the abdomen, keeping the pressure light, but increasing slightly as your hands pass over the navel. When you reach the pubic bone, fan your*

hands out and bring them very slowly up the sides of the body to the armpits. Slide your hands over the shoulders, back to the starting position. Repeat as many times as you wish, then move gently into the breast massage.

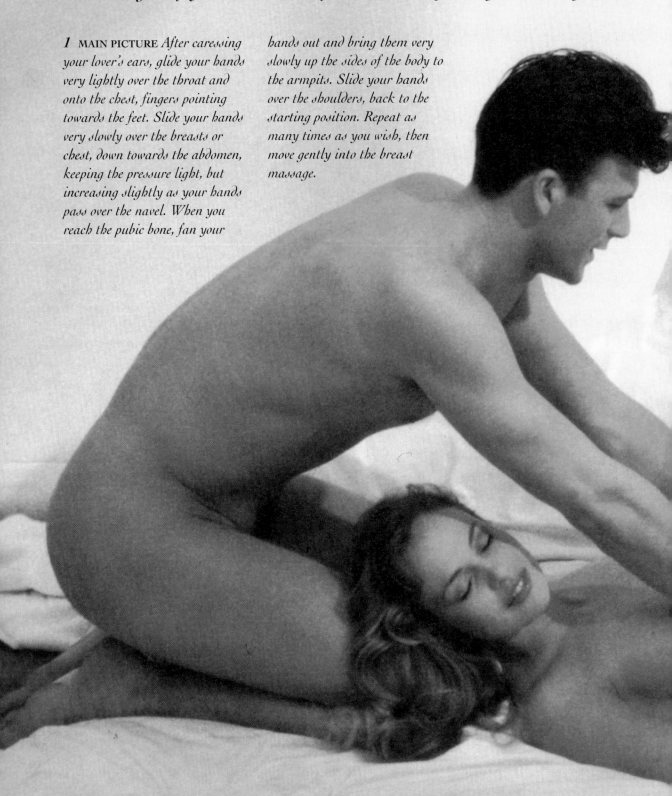

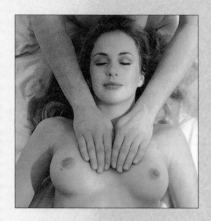

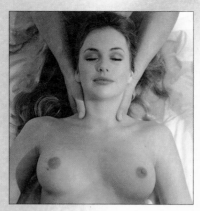

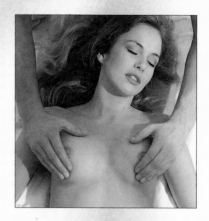

2 Place your hands on your lover's collar-bone with fingers pointing down towards the belly. Slowly and gently slide your hands down between the breasts, then around underneath them and up towards the armpits to the collar-bone. Repeat as often as desired.

3 With the tips of your fingers touching, place hands on the collar-bone. Pull your hands gently out towards the shoulders, sliding over them and up the back of the neck. Then move the starting position down and repeat the stroke towards arms, brushing lightly over the nipples.

4 Using the tips of your fingers, softly circle the nipples in ever-widening circles, avoiding direct contact with them. End this erotic stroke by gliding your hands along your lover's ribcage up toward the armpits. From here, repeat the belly slide, which is shown in step 1.

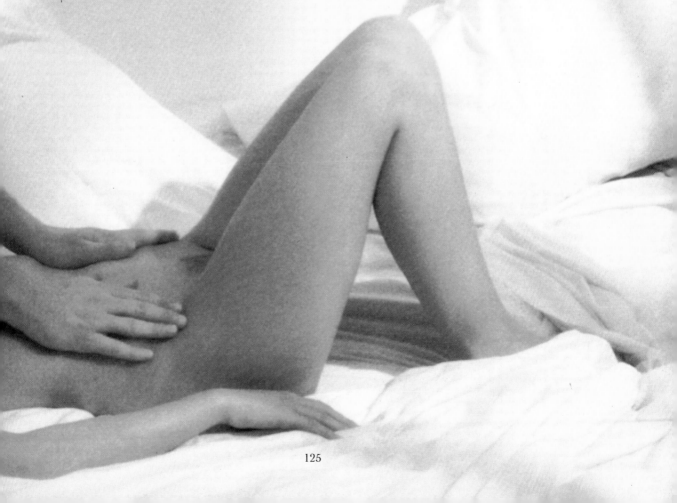

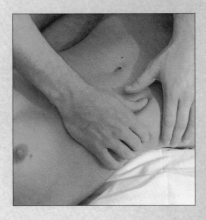

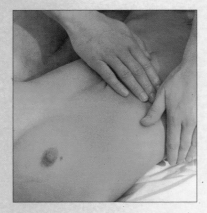

5 MAIN PICTURE *Sit to one side of your lover, then let your hands rest gently over the navel, remaining there for a few moments. Begin to massage the whole belly lightly, moving both hands, fingers and palms, clockwise around it. One hand can complete full circles, but the other will have to break contact when hands cross.*

6 ABOVE *Gently knead the waist and into the dip of the pelvis.*

7 *Do some pulling strokes up and down the waist over the hips. With your fingertips pointing downwards, gently pull each hand alternately straight up, each time overlapping the place where the last hand was. Repeat this sequence from step 5 on the other side of the waist, positioning yourself on your lover's other side.*

8 *From this position place your hands very lightly over the throat and slide them on to the chest, pulling down over the breasts/chest, towards the abdomen, keeping the pressure light but increasing slightly as your hands pass over the navel. When you reach the pubic bone, fan your hands out and slide them very slowly up the sides of the body to the armpits. Slide your hands over the shoulders, back to the starting position. This is known as the belly slide; repeat as often as you wish.*

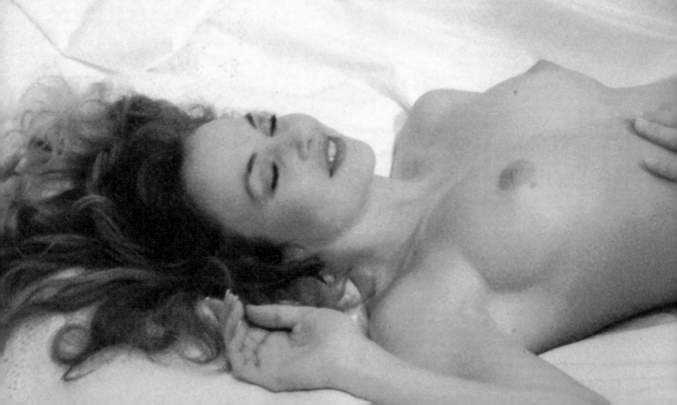

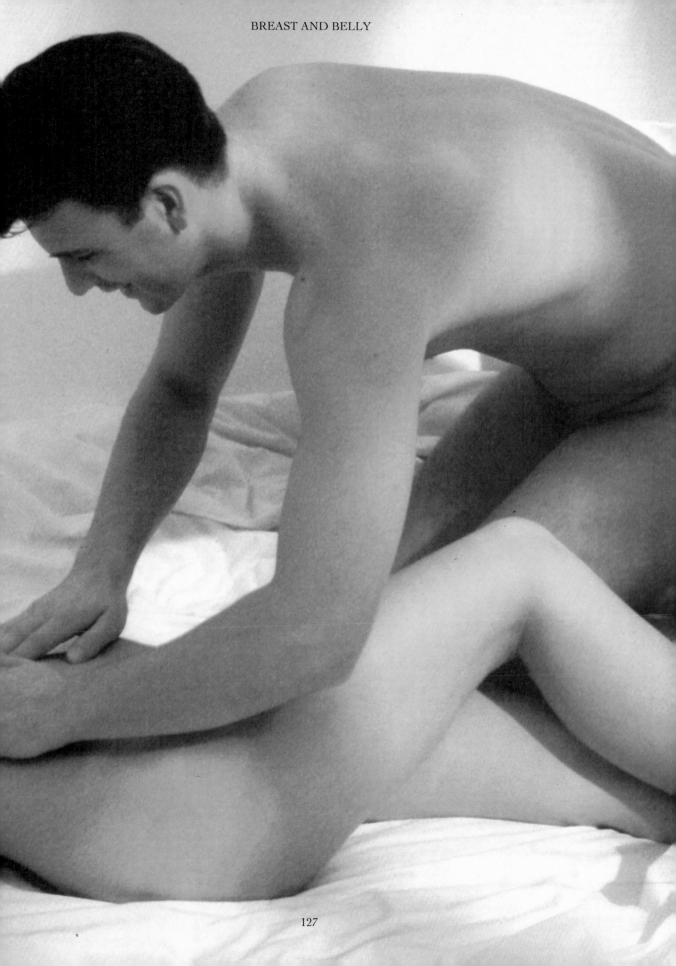

Ending the Massage

As a conclusion, do fingertip feathering downwards over the whole body from head to toes. On reaching the toes, take your hands back to the head and sweep downwards again.

1 *If you are ending on an erotic note, breathe on your lover's neck and circle the navel with your tongue. Cover the whole of your lover's body with light caresses: stroke behind the ears, touch the eyelids and lips; move around the nipples and the pubic area ... caress with your imagination!*

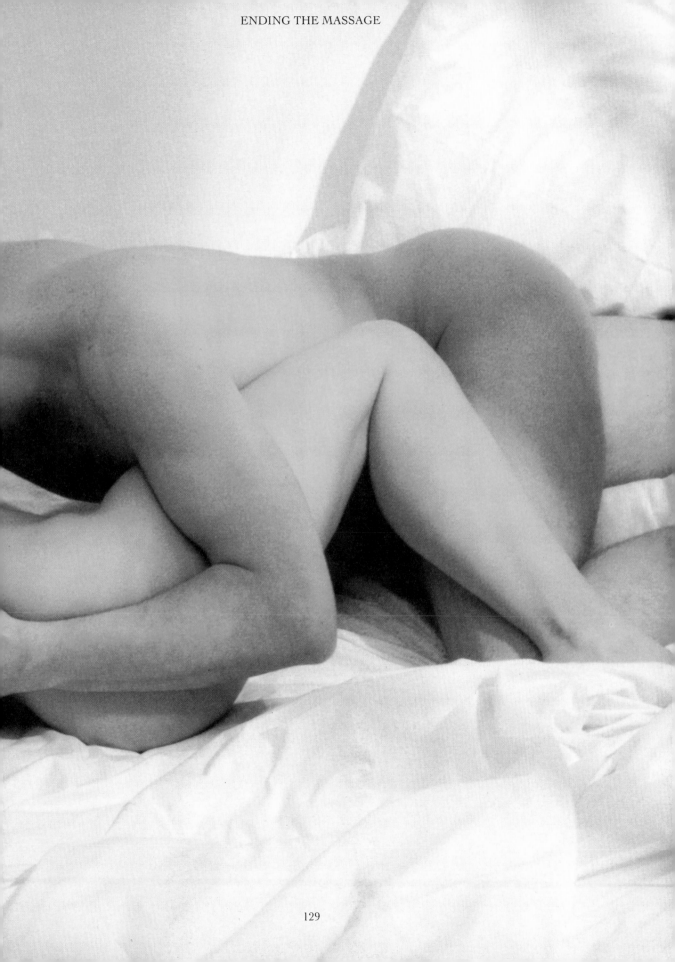

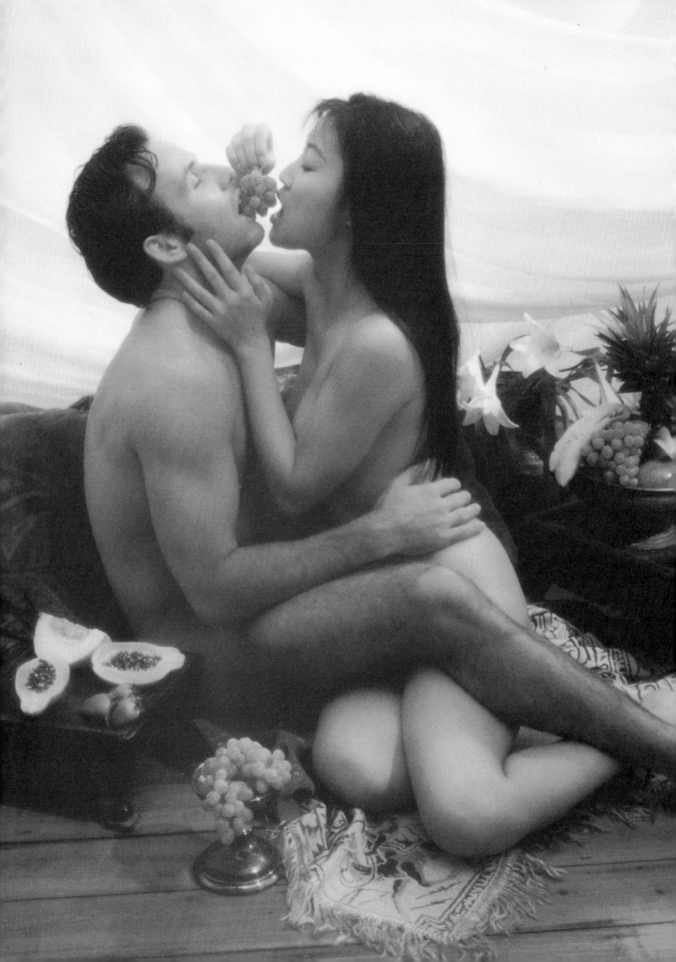

CHAPTER 8

The Food of Love

As the apple tree among the trees of the wood, so is my beloved.
I sat down under his shadow with great delight,
and his fruit was sweet to my taste.
He brought me to the banqueting house
and his banner over me was love.

The Song of Solomon

Eating for Love

You will be pleased to hear that the healthy love-food promoted in this chapter is not about raw carrots and lentils, or cholesterol and calories. Rather, it is an exploration of the safe, natural, potentially aphrodisiac foodstuffs that enhance natural body odour, heighten passion and promote a sense of well-being. Most of the foods that fall into this category are fruits, vegetables, salad greens, herbs, nuts, honey and moderate amounts of wine (between one and three glasses a day). Even chocolate has a place in this Elysian regime!

However, moderation is the keyword. No matter what chocolate manufacturers may say to the contrary, this delicacy should be regarded as an occasional treat, not a nutritious daily food in its own right. Although there is no need to avoid chocolate and other sugary goodies altogether, do take to heart the old adage 'a little of what you fancy does you good'. This is equally true in the case of wine. A little wine is felt to be beneficial to the digestion, and is also said to help lower cholesterol levels. However too much wine is bad for your liver and for your love-making!

Certainly keep moderation in mind if you plan to create a traditional dinner à *deux* as a prelude to an evening of sensual massage – you may not want to give each other a massage or make love after a heavy meal. Perhaps it is better to keep the romantic dinner as a separate sensual experience – and allow a couple of days' recovery period. But if you are determined to eat, drink and make love all night, then you will need to partake of the sustaining ambrosia of Aphrodite.

Fragrance, Food and Sensuality

By far the most comprehensive and well-researched work on the subject of sensual foods, wines and aromas is the fascinating book, *Scents and Sensuality* by the Australian researcher Max Lake. Among many other gems, Dr Lake informs us that the essential musky odour of the human male is mimicked by foods such as parsley, cooked chestnuts, parsnips and truffles. That tropical fruits such as mango and persimmon emanate a subliminal semen-like odour nuance which many women find decidedly erotic. That Champagne and camembert cheese include odour nuances that stimulate both sexes. And that chocolate contains the 'happiness chemical' phenylethlamine (PEA), and the seductive taste/aroma of vanilla, both of which promote in many people the contentment of post-coital bliss.

However, few (if any) of the aphrodisiac foodstuffs are believed to have a direct genital effect. Most have flavours, textures and/or physical characteristics that hint at sexual pleasure, either at the time of eating or several hours later when they appear in the body odour. Moreover, just like an erogenic perfume, the essential character of a 'masculine' or a 'feminine' food odour intermingles with the natural male and female essences and becomes extremely attractive. Attractive, that is, in a clean and healthy body.

Any enjoyable food can trigger a pleasurable rush, especially when we are hungry. But a few foods contain PEA – notably chocolate, as just mentioned, and also cheese. Green vegetables such as peas and green peppers are endowed with isobutyl methoxy pyraxine (IMP), a seminal flavour/odour note that many people, especially women, find delightful. The odour is also found in freshly cut grass and hay, perhaps another reason why 'love among the haystacks' is so exciting!

If this has whetted your appetite for more, see the lists on pages 135 and 136 which categorize a number of foods and beverages according to their pheromonal or mood-enhancing properties.

Nutritional Notes

The mood-enhancing effects of food are quite separate from their nutritional properties. Indeed, few nutritionists pay much attention to the subtle effects of food as explored in this chapter. It hardly seems necessary to say that maintaining a healthy diet will keep your body in good working order, and by doing so, increase your desire for an active and loving sexual relationship. It also helps you feel and look more attractive both to yourself and to your partner. So to round out the picture, let us take a brief look at the traditional indirect aids to sexual health: zinc, calcium, phosphorus and vitamin E.

Zinc is essential to the healthy functioning of the body's enzyme systems, to the healthy development of the reproductive organs and in the release of carbon dioxide. It is also said to promote male fertility by increasing sperm formation; certainly it assists in the healthy functioning of the prostate gland. Since men lose a certain amount of zinc in their semen, it would be advisable for them to ensure a good dietary source of the mineral. Zinc is also lost through sweating. Dietary sources of zinc include: oysters and other seafood, wholegrain products, pumpkin seeds, nuts, peas and beans, egg yolks, brewer's yeast and meat.

Calcium and phosphorus are the natural acid/alkali balancers of the body, helping among other things to prevent vaginal acidity and consequent irritation. Calcium forms an essential part of bones and teeth and is also necessary for blood clotting and the healthy functioning of the nervous system and muscles. Calcium-rich foods include: green leafy vegetables, yoghurt, cheese, milk, salmon and other tinned fish eaten with bones, and tofu.

Phosphorus is also essential for healthy bones and teeth, and is present along with calcium in other tissues of the body. It is necessary for the absorption of glucose and the metabolism of glucose, fat and protein. It is found mainly in dairy foods, egg yolks, wholegrain products and fish. People who 'live on their nerves' may need to boost their levels of this mineral.

The libido-increasing properties of vitamin E have not been proven. In fact, its main effect is to increase the efficiency of the heart and circulatory system. Good sources of vitamin E include: wholegrain cereals, eggs, vegetable oils, leafy greens and many other vegetables.

A big passion killer must surely be anxiety and depression. The roots of the condition can often be pinpointed to tangibles such as overwork, domestic upheaval and financial worries. But a few nutritionists such as British author Celia Wright are convinced that the food we eat affects brain chemistry and thus the way we perceive the world. She says that the first step in rebalancing body chemistry and freeing the spirit is to alkalize the blood and keep blood sugar levels up. The former can be achieved by eating plenty of fresh vegetables and fruit. Also timing of meals is important; some people need to eat little and often to achieve a state of balance. These snacks should consist of complex carbohydrate foods such as wholemeal bread, dried fruits, brown rice and wholegrain cereals.

Certain vitamins and minerals are important too. The key vitamins for both anxiety and depression are the B complex group, which help to calm and smooth the running of the nervous system. A deficiency often leads to chronic fatigue, irritability, indigestion, prematurely greying hair and skin problems. Natural sources of B complex include raw fruits and vegetables, wholegrains and brewer's yeast.

Vitamin C is also essential to help detoxify the blood and help make anti-stress hormones. It is a natural antioxidant and plays an important role in preventing premature ageing and skin wrinkling. It is found in all fresh fruits and vegetables, especially blackcurrants, citrus fruits, peppers and broccoli.

The Food of Love

Foods that Excite Men

A number of foods are said to excite men and provide an immediate rush due to the subliminal vaginal-like odour nuance which they emanate. These include foods as diverse as bean sprouts, lime, peach, oysters, hard roe and seafood in general.

Foods that Excite Women

These foods, similar to those which excite men, provide an immediate rush due to the subliminal semen-like odour nuance which they emanate. Again, it includes foods as diverse as fresh green peas, green pepper, mango, persimmon, yams and soft roe.

Foods that Excite Both Sexes

There are a number of different categories of foods which excite for different reasons. Foods which contain male and female pheromones include: camembert, caviar, oysters and unfiltered honey (*see page 132 regarding pheromones*). Some foods contain a faecal note that some people find exciting. These include: asafoetida, durian, jasmine flower tea, orange flower tea and orange flower water.

Pungent spices are all reputed aphrodisiacs due to their warming, stimulating effect. Some of the most potent include: black pepper, cinnamon, clove, coriander, cumin, fenugreek, green chillies, ginger, nutmeg and turmeric.

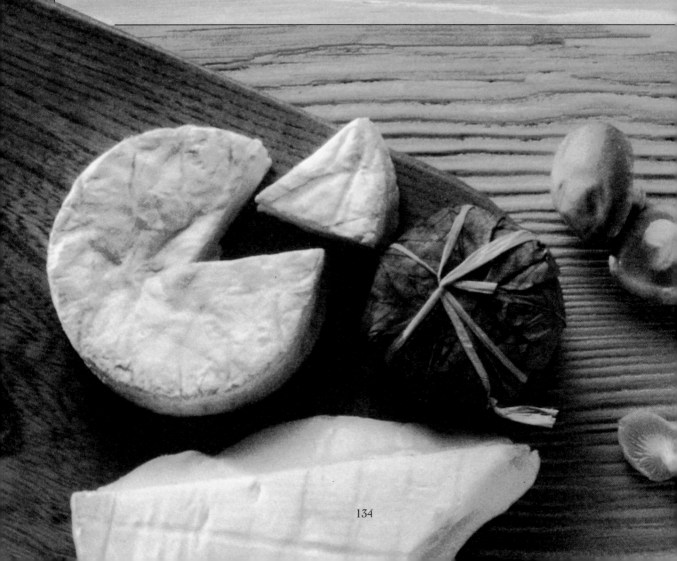

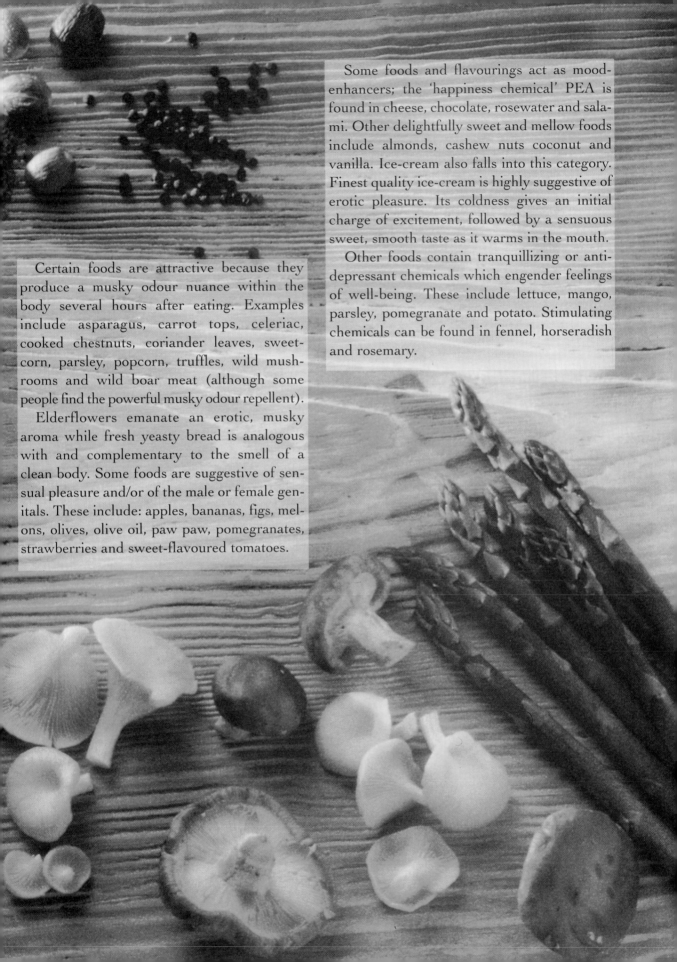

Certain foods are attractive because they produce a musky odour nuance within the body several hours after eating. Examples include asparagus, carrot tops, celeriac, cooked chestnuts, coriander leaves, sweet-corn, parsley, popcorn, truffles, wild mushrooms and wild boar meat (although some people find the powerful musky odour repellent).

Elderflowers emanate an erotic, musky aroma while fresh yeasty bread is analogous with and complementary to the smell of a clean body. Some foods are suggestive of sensual pleasure and/or of the male or female genitals. These include: apples, bananas, figs, melons, olives, olive oil, paw paw, pomegranates, strawberries and sweet-flavoured tomatoes.

Some foods and flavourings act as mood-enhancers; the 'happiness chemical' PEA is found in cheese, chocolate, rosewater and salami. Other delightfully sweet and mellow foods include almonds, cashew nuts coconut and vanilla. Ice-cream also falls into this category. Finest quality ice-cream is highly suggestive of erotic pleasure. Its coldness gives an initial charge of excitement, followed by a sensuous sweet, smooth taste as it warms in the mouth.

Other foods contain tranquillizing or anti-depressant chemicals which engender feelings of well-being. These include lettuce, mango, parsley, pomegranate and potato. Stimulating chemicals can be found in fennel, horseradish and rosemary.

An Erotic Banquet

Unless you regard cooking as a sensuous experience worth savouring, there is no need to spend many hours in the kitchen. At its simplest, a scrumptious feast for lovers could be a choice of two or three cheeses served with hot rolls and butter, celery sticks, a juicy apple or a pear, and a favourite wine. Easier still, but more stimulating, a highly aromatic Indian take-away and a bottle of good red wine. Or if you are feeling really lazy (or exceptionally amorous) just lie back and wait for the pizza delivery service to call – whatever turns you on, as they say!

But for those who are prepared to put in a little more effort, included here are a few suggestions offered by my friend Rose, sensual cook extraordinaire. She believes that sensual food is spontaneous and simple; its eroticism lies in its appeal to the senses – taste, texture, aroma, colour and aesthetic presentation. She also advocates respect for the natural essence of the food and its original environment. Equally important is the presence and awareness with which the food is eaten. If you have a garden, patio, or a balcony, what better place to share a summer lunch with your beloved?

Déjeuner au Jardin

Rose has proposed the following summer lunch menu with lovers in mind. Feel free to improvize and change the menu to suit yours and your lover's preferences.

Start with sun-warmed olives served with ciabatta bread, grilled goats' cheese and green salad and follow this with fresh deep-purple figs. Accompany your sensuous feast with a bottle of something robust and red.

Begin to prepare your feast by covering a small dish of olives (preferably the brownish, purple/black type in virgin olive-oil, not brine) with a cotton or muslin cloth, then leave out in the sun or in a sunny window to warm for an

hour or two. Prepare your leafy green salad while the olives warm in the sun.

Ciabatta bread (plain or with sun-dried tomatoes) often comes partially baked from good supermarkets and delicatessens. Just bake for fifteen minutes in a hot oven. Or buy a fully cooked ciabatta loaf from a good baker and warm through for six minutes in a moderate oven just before you wish to eat. Gently grill a round or two of creamy goats' cheese (also available from good supermarkets and delicatessens) until thoroughly cooked, then place on your previously prepared green salad.

Assemble all of the above and take into the garden or on to your balcony with a bottle of wine. Grind some green peppercorns over the cheese and salad greens, then trickle some of the olive-oil from the olive jar over the cheese, salad and ciabatta.

In full-blooded continental style, break the bread, pick up the olives with your fingers – eat them slowly to fully experience their wonderful flavour and texture. As you bite the taut skin, become aware of the soft, luscious flesh. And be aware of the rich silky oil on your fingers. Follow with the fresh figs; cut lengthways into four, then bite the exquisite fruit away from the peel. Gently inhale the symphony of aromas, the spice aroma of newly-crushed green peppercorns, the ciabatta, the olives, the faint muskiness of the warm cheese and the delicate sweetness of the figs ... ecstacy!

Incidentally, although this is an ideal summer lunch, try bringing the warmth of summer to a cold winter's day – or night. Prepare as above, but warm the olives through in a covered oven-proof dish on the bottom shelf of the oven. Fresh figs may be impossible to obtain in the winter, so finish with whatever sensual fruit you can find – mango would be an especially good alternative. Assemble as for the garden but take to bed.

A Sumptuous Supper

A sumptuous supper for two may sound like a great deal of work, but you need not spend hours in the kitchen to create a meal filled with visual and sensual delight. The suggested menu includes ciabatta bread pizza, a green salad with nasturtium flowers (if in season), a wonderful wine of your choice, followed by pears poached in elderflower cordial and vanilla and later, cardamom coffee or aromatic tea (*see page 143*).

Cut a ciabatta loaf lengthways and brush with olive-oil. Spread with some home-made fresh tomato sauce, then pile the bread with a few of the following toppings: mozzarella slices or goats' cheese, sun-dried tomatoes bottled in olive-oil, garlic, olives, capers bottled in brine not vinegar, baby artichokes bottled in oil, spanish onion slices, peppers, mushrooms and fresh chopped basil or oregano. Trickle a little olive-oil over the pizza and bake in a moderate oven for about fifteen minutes. Finally brown under the grill for a minute or two.

While the pizza is in the oven prepare a crisp green salad brightened with a few nasturtium flowers if they are in season. For the salad dressing, mix together a tablespoon of lemon or lime juice (and half a teaspoon of grated zest if you wish), three tablespoons of extra-virgin olive-oil, half a teaspoon of runny honey, a seasoning of freshly milled green or black peppercorns and a little sea salt. Do not dress the salad until just before you are ready to eat.

Before you begin the main course, prepare the elderflower pears. Halve two firm pears and put them in a casserole dish. You can either remove the peel or leave it on, but do leave the stems attached. Add a couple of tablespoons of water, two dessertspoons of elderflower cordial and a vanilla pod. Cover the dish and cook in a moderate oven for about thirty minutes or until the pears are soft. Remove the vanilla pod, drain off any excess juice, then sprinkle with chopped toasted almonds or hazelnuts then serve with some whipped cream.

If you or your lover adores chocolate then this chocolate and chestnut dessert may be a good alternative. Put 3 fl oz/ 90 ml of chestnut puree into a mixing bowl then add 4 oz/125 g of melted dark chocolate and a dessertspoon of brandy to the puree and mix. Add a little runny honey according to taste and a few drops of natural vanilla extract. Fold in 4 fl oz/100 ml of strained Greek yoghurt or double cream if you prefer. Pour into two attractive dishes and decorate with a sprinkling of chopped *marron glacés* (glazed chestnuts available from delicatessens) and a few crystallized flowers. Chill for an hour then serve with cream.

Crystallized flowers are expensive to buy, yet easy to make at home. The most beautiful of the edible flowers are violets, roses, primroses, flowering cherry and apple blossom. Pick the best-looking flowers on a warm dry day when there is no rain or dew on the petals. Make a syrup of 1 lb/450 g of sugar and 16 fl oz/480 ml of water and boil for five minutes. Drop the flower heads or petals into the syrup and boil for one minute. Using a slotted spoon remove the flowers from the syrup and place on a baking sheet lined with greaseproof or waxed paper. Leave in a warm dry place for one or two days until dry and hard. Once dry store in a glass jar with a tight-fitting lid.

Flowers and Essences

For a summertime feast, scatter a few rose or geranium petals over the tablecloth. When fresh flowers are not available, strew dried flower heads across the cloth to soften a too-formal table setting, thus imparting a sense of abandoned rapture. Burn candles perfumed with floral or spicy essential oils (*see page 83*) or vaporize rosewater or orange flower water in a diffuser, made more fragrant with a few drops of geranium, ylang ylang, petitgrain, rose or sandalwood essential oil.

Sensual Wines

No erotic feast would seem complete without wine. As old as civilization itself, wine has always been an integral part of celebration and feasting. There are references to it in ancient Egyptian paintings and we know that the Greeks and Romans loved wine.

It had a significant part to play in the religious rites and ceremonies of many cultures throughout the world, and it continues to occupy that role in many countries today.

But we also know that wine is a drink favoured by lovers, ancient and modern. A sensible quantity of wine is a marvellous aphrodisiac for both sexes, tantalizing the senses, and triggering an immediate 'happiness chemical' rush. It combines colour, bouquet, taste, subliminal pain (if sparkling or very dry), and the effect of the alcohol itself – a lessening of inhibitions. As if this were not enough, good wine also contains an appreciable quantity of sexy grape pheromones – what more could you ask of an aphrodisiac?

There are a number of wines which have specific effects, notably scenting the body after consumption. The following information may help you choose a sensual wine to accompany your love-feast.

Wine made from the red grape cabernet sauvignon scents the whole body within six hours of drinking. These small tough-skinned grapes are found in the red wines of Bordeaux. Many Australian, Chilean, South African and Californian wines are also produced using this fragrant and distinctive grape.

Any wine (red or white) that has been aged in oak barrels produces an erotic musky odour nuance. Apparently the wine picks up certain characteristics from the wood, including extra

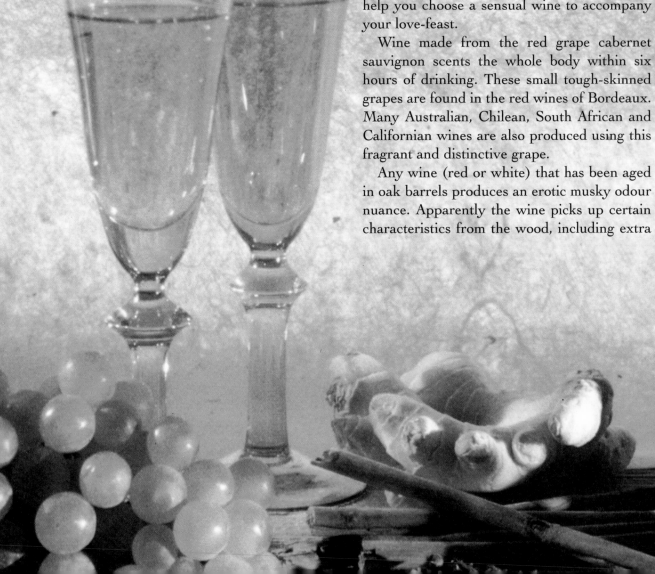

tannin and vanillin, giving it an intoxicating vanilla flavour. The aging action of oxygen on the wine in oak barrels is also thought to be of some significance.

Wine produced from shiraz (or sirah) grapes produces a musky odour nuance very similar to that of cabernet sauvignon. Look for wines produced in California and Australia for this particular grape.

Champagne must surely be the favourite wine for lovers, as well as being a necessary item on most celebration menus; weddings and christening wouldn't be the same without it. Although it is expensive when compared with other wines, for a very special lovers' feast, nothing else will do. These days it is possible to buy a very decent Champagne for a reasonable price from most good supermarkets. According to experts, it is not necessary to serve Champagne icy cold; simply cool well and drink!

Along with its incomparable taste, Champagne contains seductive 'sweaty' and 'yeasty' notes derived from the pinot noir and chardonnay grapes from which it is made. A number of cheaper white wines produced from chardonnay, semillon and riesling grapes also contain these 'sweaty' and 'yeasty' notes without the enchanting bubbles found in Champagne But any wine drunk in the company of a loving partner will take on the delightful headiness of the most expensive Champagne, regardless of the colour, cost or vintage.

But you are not confined to conventional wines if your fancy takes you elsewhere. Mead or honey-wine – buzzing with flower and grape pheromones – is the classic aphrodisiac for those who can enjoy its incredible sweetness. In Saxon times newlyweds drank it for a month after the wedding ceremony (the 'honeymoon' period) to sustain sexual desire and stamina. Mead also makes an excellent mulled wine, perhaps made less sweet with plenty of lemon or lime, and pungent whole spices such as cloves, pieces of cinnamon stick and ginger root. Home-made elderflower wine gives an immediate erotic charge due to the musky aroma of the flowers.

But what about beer? Hops contain oestrogenic substances which apart from being soporific, act to dampen the male libido. So a small quantity of beer is a great mood-enhancer for women, but macho beer-drinking men beware! The phytohormones in hops may contribute to laying down extra fat, especially around the belly – somewhat akin to a pseudo-pregnancy.

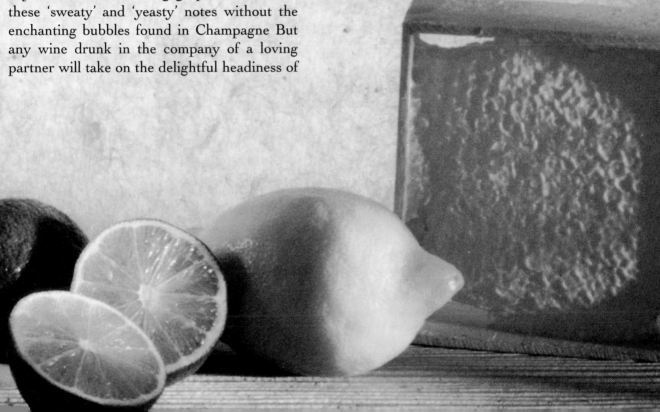

Sensual Fruit

Fruit is one of the most sensuous and flavourful and healthy groups of food available to us. It is also one of the most diverse groups of foods offering a fabulous range of fragrance, taste and texture. Make room for some in your sensuous feast menu and with your lover, savour the textures, enjoy the aromas, revel in the fresh tastes and sensations.

Don't save fruit for the table – take to bed any sensual fruit you fancy – fresh figs or a wonderfully aromatic and ripe mango would be absolutely perfect.

Pleasure yourself and your lover with a bowl of musky sun-warmed raspberries or delight in lychees individually peeled. Pull the creamy white flesh with its sudden tang from the stone by your teeth and pass it from your own lips into the eager mouth of your lover.

Eat strawberries from the stalk – just as they are in midsummer, or marinated in Cointreau and a little honey later in the season.

In winter, savour baked apples cooked with butter, honey and chopped hazelnuts.

Indulge yourself and luxuriate in an aromatic bath with a glass of mulled wine and dish of fresh lychees – and dream of your lover.

Relish the juicy flesh of melon complimented with the pungent aroma of ginger. Simply sprinkle the fruit with a tiny amount of the finely grated, fresh root.

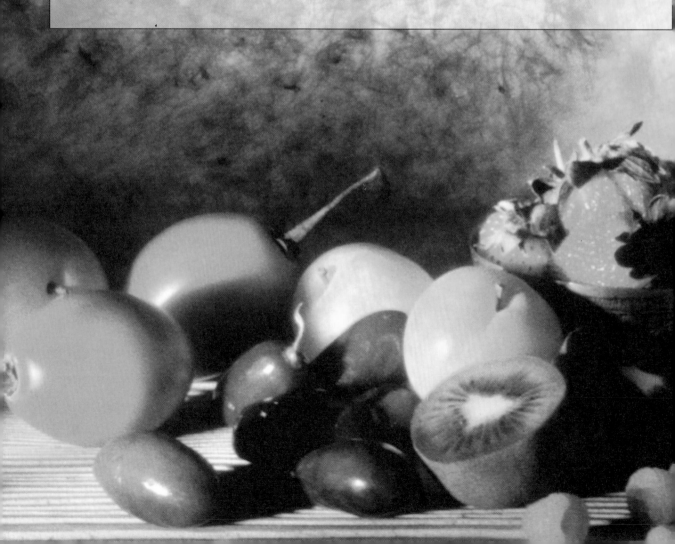

A Romantic Fruit Salad

There is probably nothing quite as fragrantly sensual as fruit salad. Indulge yourself and your lover with this delicious and exotic treat by marinading slices of star fruit in a little chablis (white wine made from chardonnay grapes) for about half an hour. Add sliced pear, halved and de-seeded green grapes and a little more wine. Leave for another fifteen minutes. Carefully mix in strawberry halves, blueberries and, very carefully so as not to squash them, some raspberries. Cover the bowl and allow the aromas to intermingle for up to an hour before serving. A little honey may be added in the early stages if you wish. For a subtle, but very distinctive flavour, heat the seeds of two cardamom pods with the chablis and use as a marinade. Remove the seeds by pouring the wine through a fine mesh sieve.

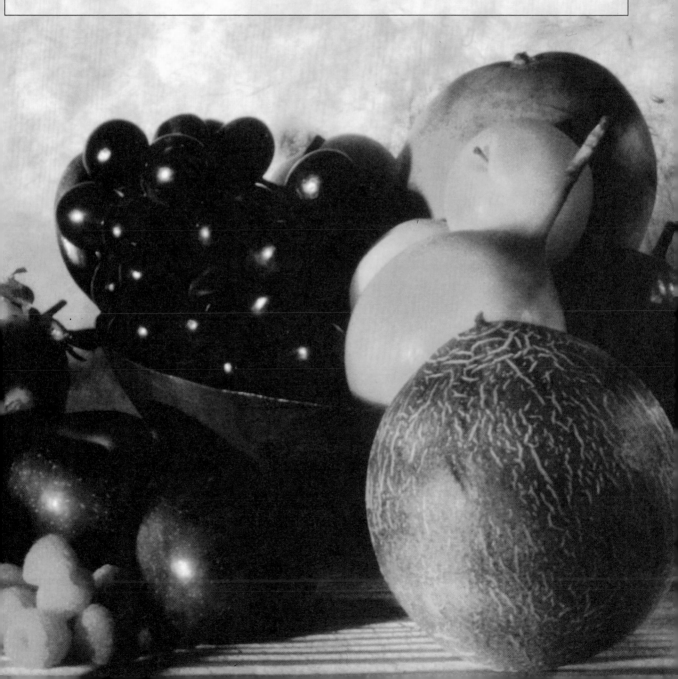

Sweet Seductions

End your sumptuous love-feast with a beautifully fragrant treat which can be served at the end of a meal, or eaten as a snack in bed. If you live in a large city then these goodies (and many others) can be obtained from ethnic grocers or delicatessens.

Try real Turkish delight flavoured with rose-water – a taste of eastern heaven. Or baklava – a delicious Middle Eastern light-as-air pastry filled with almonds and pistachio nuts and sweetened with honey.

Another delicious treat is rashmali, a chilled Indian sweetmeat made from milk curds, rose-water and pistachio nuts. As well as tasting divine, it helps to sweeten the breath and settle the stomach – especially good after a curry.

Halva, a delectable sweetmeat from Greece, made from tahini (ground sesame seeds), honey and pistachios, is another possibility.

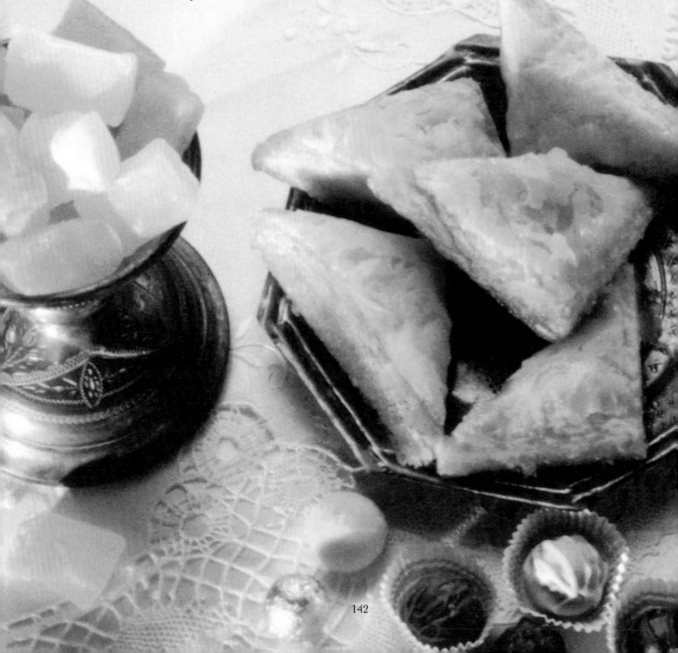

Cardamom Coffee

Add half a teaspoon of ground cardamom spice to every two dessertspoons of freshly ground coffee and make in the usual way. Cardamom coffee is usually taken black in the Middle East, with a little sugar or honey to taste. The spice acts to buffer the harsh effects on the stomach associated with drinking black coffee. As well as sweetening the breath, cardamom aids the digestion of rich food.

Aromatic Tea

Alternatively, drink Indian tea without milk, flavoured with mint or lemon balm. Put about a half ounce/12 g of the fresh herb (or a teaspoon of dried mint or lemon balm) into the teapot with the usual amount of Indian tea. Allow to brew for six minutes before pouring. Mint and lemon balm, like cardamom, sweeten the breath, buffer the harsh effects of black tea, and aid the digestion of rich food. Should you prefer to avoid caffeine, make straight peppermint, spearmint or lemon balm tea.

Breakfast In Bed

As romantic as dinner *à deux*, breakfast in bed can be an enchanting and indulgent way to start your lover's day. Bring your lover a glass of Bucks Fizz (Champagne, mango or orange juice and a splash of brandy), served with warm croissants (or wholegrain toast), butter and a choice of three different types of honey such as heather, acacia and Tasmanian forest. For a cheaper version of Bucks Fizz, use sparkling wine instead of real Champagne, and leave out the brandy. Or you may prefer to drink a fine Indian or China tea such as Assam, Earl Grey or Lapsang – or a stimulating cup of Viennese coffee (flavoured with roasted figs). Bon appetit!

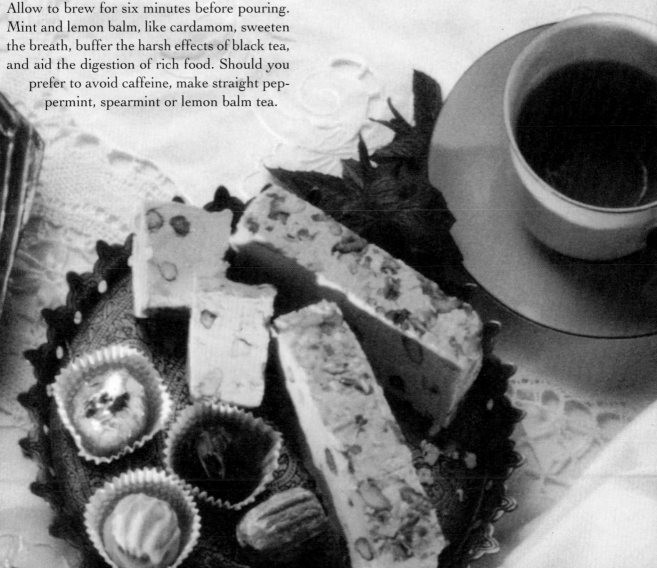

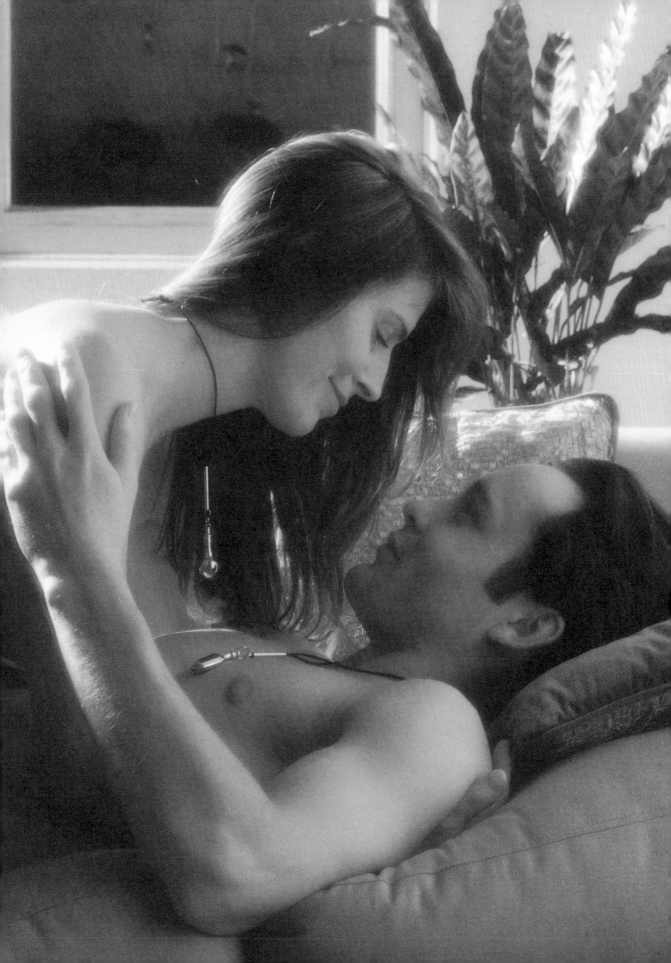

CHAPTER 9

A Fragrant Talisman

Fragrance may well be the signature of eternity.

Tom Robbins

Making a Love Potion

Just as lovers may have their special tune, aromatherapy lovers have their magical fragrance – a sacred love potion which acts on the deep psyche, recalling the joys of making love together in the perfumed garden of Aphrodite. Put several drops of your partner's favourite aromatic blend on a new handkerchief. Whenever you are away from each other, a mere whiff will summon up the presence of your beloved. Likewise, your lover could carry a remnant of your own personal blend. Each time you inhale the fragrance, a rush of loving sensations will flood your whole being and create a fragrant link between your hearts.

When preparing the fragrant talisman, it is important to work together; to regard it as an act of love. You can use a massage oil blend as a love token, or you may prefer to make a concentrated essential oil perfume or aromatic water. Having created your own personal blend – the fragrance that your partner associates with you – exchange the oils with love.

However, it is not enough to throw together your lover's favourite blend in their absence and to use this as a fragrant reminder. It is vital that your partner mixes their own blend of oils – and vice versa, otherwise the essence of your beloved will be missing. Believe it or not, no two people can blend an identical-smelling fragrance, even though they may use exactly the same blend of oils in exactly the same quantities from the same bottles. Amazingly, the oil will always take on an aspect of the blender's personality – their aromatic signature. Moreover, a massage oil or perfume blended while you are feeling depressed, angry or distressed, will not smell right, no matter how beautiful the ingredients. It may smell rather flat, murky or somewhat harsh. On the other hand, a perfume blended with loving thoughts will be especially vibrant.

But don't take my word for it. Get together a group of three or four friends – preferably of widely differing personalities – then prepare an identical aromatherapy blend, say, 2 drops of lavender, 2 drops of geranium and 1 drop of patchouli, in a 10 ml bottle of base oil. Each person should label their own blend with their name, then hold the bottle for at least five minutes in order for the oil to become imbibed with their personal 'vibes'. Once everyone has completed the task, compare aromas. I think you will be surprised!

Although I have used the terms 'love potion', 'love philtre' and 'aphrodisiac' synonymously, they are quite different. An aphrodisiac acts in a purely physiological way, whereas a love potion or philtre is supposed to act through magical forces. However, when it comes to the use of aromatics, it becomes difficult to separate the physical from the psychological.

There is also a difference between a talisman and an amulet, although the two are often confused. An amulet is mostly protective and is supposed to deflect bad influences. A talisman, on the other hand, is a magical object charged with the actual force it is meant to represent. So a fragrant talisman is both a material and a spiritual link between you and your lover, and will go on working for you as long as the relationship remains sweet.

Perfume-making

Commercial perfumes are usually suspended in ethyl alcohol – labelled 'ethanol' – but this is not generally available in Britain without a perfumier's licence. Moreover, alcohol is very drying to the skin. For this reason, aromatherapists tend to favour the oil or beeswax-based perfumes which have the advantage of lingering on the skin for much longer. Essential oils can also be partially suspended in distilled water or floral water to form very good aromatic waters or aftershave formulas.

Oil-based Perfumes

Oil-based perfumes have been used in the making of charms and love potions since antiquity. To the weaver of enchantment, the full moon is the most auspicious time for spell-casting. For just as the moon influences the ebb and flow of the tides, she is said to influence the ebb and flow of the emotions.

Fill a 10 ml dark glass bottle almost to the top with jojoba, light coconut oil or infused oil of vanilla (*see below*). Build your perfume blend slowly, drop by drop, shaking after each addition and smelling as you go. You will need between 15 and 20 drops altogether.

Once mixed, leave your perfume for a few weeks to mature. Keep in a cool dark place, but shake the bottle once a day to facilitate the process. At the end of the maturation period, the blend will have lost its 'raw' overtone and will smell much more rounded. An oil-based perfume will keep for about six months if kept away from heat and light.

Infused Oil of Vanilla

Vanilla oil makes a beautifully sensual base for a love potion, perfume or erotic massage oil.

Incidentally, it was the sixteenth-century Spanish explorer Cortez who introduced vanilla to Europe. He discovered it in Mexico, where the Aztecs used it to flavour their chocolate drinks. The combination of chocolate and vanilla was deemed so arousing that Aztec women were forbidden the pleasure!

Unfortunately, infused oil of vanilla needs to be prepared at least a month in advance. So if you delight in this soulful aroma, make plenty of it for future use.

You will need 50 ml of light coconut oil or jojoba, a vanilla pod and a clear glass jar with a tight fitting lid. Simply split the vanilla pod down the middle, then cut into little pieces and put in the jar. Cover with the oil, then leave the tightly sealed jar outside in the sun (or on a warm radiator or boiler) for about five weeks, bringing the jar indoors at night. Give the jar a good shake every time you pass by to facilitate the process of infusion. After five weeks or when the oil smells fragrant enough for your taste, strain the mixture through muslin and store in a dark glass bottle. The oil will keep for at least a year.

Oil-based Love Potions

Each of the potions below specifies the number of drops required to each 10 ml of base oil. Coconut oil tends to be somewhat cheaper than jojoba oil.

Shiva		Shakti		King Solomon		Queen of Sheba	
OIL	DROPS	OIL	DROPS	OIL	DROPS	OIL	DROPS
Black pepper	5	Bergamot	3	Frankincense	5	Bergamot	6
Lime	3	Coriander	3	Ginger	1	Jasmine	4
Sandalwood	10	Geranium	3	Lemon	6	Coriander	6
Ylang ylang	5	Rose	3	Ylang lang	5	Lavender	3
Light coconut oil or jojoba, or infused oil of vanilla	10 ml	Ylang ylang	6	Jojoba or light coconut oil	10 ml	Infused oil of vanilla	10 ml
		Infused oil of vanilla	10 ml				

Beeswax Perfumes

The ancients of Egypt, Greece and Rome favoured a mixture of animal fat and heavy vegetable oils such as olive or castor as a carrier for their perfumed unguents. The resulting mixtures containing extracts of woods, spices, flowers and resins were used to perfume the whole body, including the soles of the feet. It is said that Cleopatra's favourite perfume was cyprinum, a heady concoction containing oil of henna flowers.

The perfumes and cosmetics so popular with the Greeks soon became fashionable in Rome. The Roman historian Pliny describes a costly unguent called susinum, which originated in Athens. He tells us it was composed of extracts of white lilies, roses, saffron and myrrh.

If, like the ancients, you would prefer a solid perfume, but unlike them you do not wish to incorporate animal fat, honey-scented beeswax is a wonderful alternative. It also imparts its own subtle fragrance to the blend. Moreover, you could use infused oil of vanilla to soften the beeswax instead of plain jojoba or coconut oil. Try one of the formulas suggested here, or perhaps use a single essence such as rose, sandalwood, jasmine, neroli or ylang ylang to perfume the beeswax base. Due to the high concentration of essential oil, this perfume will keep for up to six months if stored in a tightly covered container in a cool dark place.

Ingredients

1 rounded teaspoon of grated beeswax
2 teaspoons (10 ml) of jojoba or coconut oil or infused oil of vanilla
20-25 drops of essential oil

Method

Blend the essential oils with the jojoba, coconut oil or infused oil of vanilla. Carefully melt the beeswax in a small heatproof bowl placed over a milk saucepan of simmering water. Remove from the heat and stir in your already prepared perfume blend. Pour into a small sterilized glass pot, cover tightly and label. Wax perfume does not take a long time to ripen and can be used within one or two days after it has been made.

How to Apply Oil or Beeswax Perfumes

Perfume is usually applied to the pulse points – behind the ears, the sides of the neck, the inside of the wrists, the elbow creases, behind the knees and around the ankles. Apparently, as well as being erogenous zones, these pulse points help to radiate the fragrance because they are fractionally warmer than other skin areas. Moreover, there are those who would swear that perfume smells better when applied to these special places.

Beeswax Love Potions

Each of the potions below specifies a number of drops to 10 ml of base oil and 1 teaspoon of grated beeswax. Follow the basic method outlined above.

Honeydew		Honeymoon		Aphrodite's Nectar		Bee-witched	
OIL	DROPS	OIL	DROPS	OIL	DROPS	OIL	DROPS
Rose	5	Patchouli	10	Bergamot	5	Bergamot	5
Sandalwood	10	Ylang ylang	10	Jasmine	10	Clary sage	5
Ylang ylang	5			Petitgrain	5	Rose	10

Aromatic Waters

Despite a preference for heavy oil-based perfumes, floral waters were not unknown in the ancient world. Indeed, lavender water was one of the first to be prepared by the Romans. In the tenth century AD, the Persian physician Avicenna began to obtain floral waters by a distillation process and the use of rosewater in particular, became an all-consuming passion. Rosewater and other 'perfumes of Arabia' were brought back to Europe by crusading knights, along with the knowledge of distillation.

Napoleon's final exile to St Helena after his defeat at Waterloo took him permanently away from Paris, parting him from his perfumier, Chardin. No longer could he indulge his passion for the rosemary-based cologne that reminded him of his childhood in Corsica, where rosemary grew wild in the underbrush of the *maquis*.

To make your own aromatic water, fill a 100 ml dark glass bottle with distilled water, orange flower water or rosewater, or a 50/50 mixture of floral waters. Build the fragrance gradually by adding a few drops of essential oil at a time, shaking the bottle and smelling as you go. Add up to 100 drops of essential oil in all, which is the average strength for most colognes. Then allow the mixture to ripen for a few weeks before use. Keep in a cool dark place, but remember to shake well each day as you pass by to facilitate the process of infusion. When ready, pour through a damp coffee-filter paper, rebottle and label. For best results, funnel into a perfume atomizer before use.

Should you prefer not to filter the blend (after all, a great deal of essential oil will be left behind on the filter paper), you will need to shake the bottle (or atomizer) each time before use to disperse the oils.

How to Apply an Aromatic Water

These can be used in the same way as commercial products – splashed on after a bath or shower, brushed through the hair or sprinkled over clothes. However, the best way to apply an aromatic water is to spray it on using a perfume atomizer.

Aromatic Water Love Potions

Each blend below specifies a number of drops to each 100 ml of floral water. Water-based perfumes can be made in larger quantities because they are used more liberally.

Woodland Rapture		Nuance		Blue Lagoon		Salome	
OIL	DROPS	OIL	DROPS	OIL	DROPS	OIL	DROPS
Clary sage	20	Bergamot	40	Bergamot	20	Bergamot	35
Elemi	3	Clary sage	20	Clary sage	10	Cardamom	2
Cedarwood	20	Geranium	10	Lavender	25	Grapefruit	10
Juniper	20	Neroli	15	Lemon	10	Lavender	20
Petitgrain	30	Patchouli	10	Lime	5	Orange	20
Vetiver	5	Rosewater	100 ml	Petitgrain	20	Rose	8
Orange flower				Rosemary	10	Orange flower	
water	100 ml			Distilled		water	50 ml
				water	100 ml	Rosewater	50 ml

Aftershave Formulas

At most periods in history men have used perfume without being thought of as unmanly. Indeed, it is far stranger that the habit was ever lost. It was the Victorians who deemed that a 'real' man should smell only of tobacco, tweed and beer – a notion that still lingers among many dyed-in-the-wool traditionalists. However, even the most conservative of men these days may be tempted by a gently antiseptic, yet seductively aromatic aftershave formula. Commercial products usually contain a high concentration of alcohol and synthetic fragrance which can irritate the sensitive skin of the face. Therefore, the simple aromatic aftershave formulas suggested here are alcohol-free. Instead, they contain a small quantity of cider vinegar which helps to restore the skin's natural acid/alkali balance.

Making Aftershave Formulas

Pour 300 ml of rosewater, orange flower water, or distilled water into a dark glass bottle. Add 1 or 2 teaspoons of cider vinegar and shake well. Then add between 3 and 5 drops of essential oil or combination of oils. The aftershave formula is then ready to use. There is no need to filter the blend, but do remember to shake the bottle each time before use in order to disperse the oils once again.

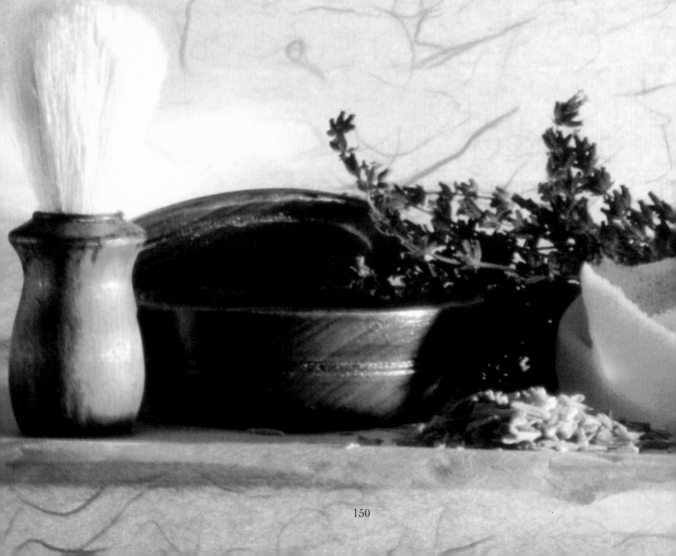

Seductive Aftershave Formulas

Each of the aftershave formulas below specifies the number of drops to
each 300 ml of floral water and 2 teaspoons of cider vinegar.

Panther

OIL	DROPS
Coriander	2
Sandalwood	2
Vetiver	1

Night Flight

OIL	DROPS
Cedarwood	1
Clary sage	1
Patchouli	2

Kama Sutra

OIL	DROPS
Bergamot	2
Frankincense	2
Rose	1

Ananga Ranga

OIL	DROPS
Coriander	1
Sandalwood	2
Ylang ylang	2

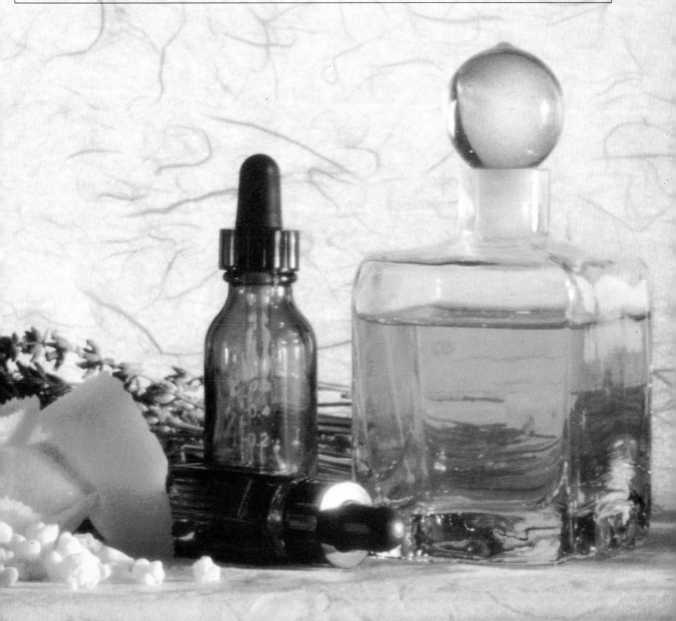

Afterword

Led by the enigmatic sense of smell, this book has been a journey through the senses. Yet far from advocating sensory stimulation for its own sake, the aim has been to awaken in our hearts the capacity to experience the sensation of joy. In so doing, we radiate this feeling to others in our sphere, not just to the person with whom we share a sexual relationship.

Indeed, the practice of sensual aroma-therapy does more than stimulate the erogenous zones. As well as being a beautiful and pleasurable way to nurture a loving relationship, it is a path towards deeper fulfilment, a path which leads to the ultimate goal of self-acceptance. However this does not mean that we must struggle to be perfect before we can be comfortable with ourselves. Such a monumental task will only succeed in creating further tension and conflict. Instead, our purpose is to learn to live life to the full, to be loving and true to ourselves. It is through the spirit of playfulness, spontaneity, creativity and relaxation that we enhance our physical and emotional well-being – and our life as a whole.

Appendix
Useful Equipment

You will need a supply of dark glass bottles and jars with screw-top lids – these are available in various sizes from pharmacies or from specialist shops selling home-made cosmetic materials and herbs. Alternatively, recycle any suitable glass bottles and jars, but do not use plastic bottles. Essential oils tend to react with plastic, especially if in contact with the substance for any length of time.

Other useful items include:
- Coffee-filter papers for filtering water-based blends
- Heat-resistant glass or pottery bowl which will fit over a small saucepan of simmering water (the *bain marie* method), used for melting beeswax in the making of solid perfumes
- Glass measuring jug and small funnel
- Kitchen grater suitable for grating beeswax
- Muslin for straining aromatic decoctions prepared from whole spices
- Palette knife, teaspoon, dessertspoon, tablespoon
- Plastic 5 ml measuring spoon for measuring small quantities of base oil (widely available from pharmacies, chemists or drug stores)
- Self-adhesive labels for labelling your aromatic concoctions
- Spirit pen – ideal for writing on labels as the ink is smudge-proof

---

Weights and Measures

For the benefit of American readers, the following conversion table may be helpful.

Liquid Measure (dry if appropriate)

1 teaspoon = 5 ml

3 teaspoons = 1 tablespoon = 15 ml

2 tablespoons = 1 fl oz = 30 ml

1 cup = 8 fl oz = 0.24 litre (240 ml)

2 cups = 1 pint = 0.47 litre

4 cups = 1 quart = 0.95 litre

Weight

1oz = 28 g

1 lb = 454 g

1 lb = 0.45 kg

Please consult your local retailers and Yellow Pages for information on the availability of essential oils and on training courses.

Glossary

Absolute A highly concentrated aromatic oil extracted from plant material, usually flowers, by volatile solvents such as hexane and petroleum ether.

Androstenone The principal male pheromone produced by the apocrine glands in the skin. However, it is formed in both sexes by the influence of testosterone. It drives the menstrual cycle and is the raw fuel of the libido of both sexes.

Aphrodisiac Derived from the Greek *aphrodisios*, belonging to Aphrodite, the goddess of love. A drug, food or massage oil with the power to increase sexual desire and to enhance sexual performance.

Aromatherapy The therapeutic use of essential oils.

Carrier/base oil A vegetable oil such as almond or grapeseed in which essential oils are diluted for massage.

Concrete A concentrated waxy, solid or semi-solid perfume material; a by-product of volatile solvent extraction used to obtain an absolute.

Copulins Highly volatile female pheromones occurring in the genitals, rising to a peak at ovulation.

Distillation The process of evaporating a liquid and condensing its vapour. The classic method for obtaining plant essences.

Effleurage From the French, meaning to stroke. The simplest and most instinctive of all the massage strokes.

Endorphin (also enkephalin, beta endorphin, casomorphin and dynorphin) A morphine-like family of molecules produced in body cells, especially in parts of the brain and spinal cord. They block pain and 'lift' mood. Feelings of relaxation and/or joy raise the level of these 'happiness chemicals'.

Essential oil/essence The odoriferous volatile (evaporates in the open air) component of an aromatic plant, usually captured by distillation or expression (see also ethereal oil, volatile oil).

Ethereal oil Another term for essential oil. An apt description because plant essences quickly evaporate into the ether.

Expression A method used for capturing the essential oils of citrus fruits. The oil is found in the outer rind and is obtained by pressure. Although this was once carried out by hand, machines using centrifugal force are now used instead.

Feathering Very light, fingertip massage stroke, applied with a sweeping action.

Fixed oil Ordinary vegetable oil such as olive or almond which, unlike an essential oil, does not evaporate in the open air.

Friction A massage stroke which uses the ball of the thumb, fingers or heel of the hand to apply moderate pressure in a circular motion.

Hormone According to the classical definition, a chemical secreted in the blood which acts on cells elsewhere in the body. However, the most recent definition is a chemical secreted by body cells (including brain cells) which diffuses into the body fluids to act on other cells both nearby and distant.

Infused oil Usually a herbal oil such as marigold (*calendula*) or St John's Wort (*hypericum*). Plant material is placed in vegetable oil and heated until the aroma has permeated the oil. It is then strained and used as a massage oil or healing agent for skin complaints.

IMP (isomethoxy propyl pyrezine) The principal odour nuance of green vegetables, especially fresh green peas and green peppers. Believed to have a subthreshold seminal odour, especially attractive to women.

Indole A foul-smelling odour found in the rear end of animals and their waste products. Also found in infinitesimal quantities in certain flowers such as jasmine, neroli and lilac. Said to be sexually stimulating for both sexes, but only at subthreshold levels.

IVA (isovaleric acid) Present in the healthy vagina as a result of the action of lactic acid bacteria. Also found in certain cheeses, especially brie and camembert.

Limbic system Originally called the 'smell brain'. Extends from the midbrain into the base of the neo-cortex. As well as odour perception, it deals with visceral activity such as sexual feelings, intuition, creativity, emotions and probably much more besides. The limbic system is little understood and remains a subject of ongoing research.

Oestrogen One of the female hormones synthesized in the ovaries and by cells in the cortex of the adrenal glands. Also secreted in the adrenals of males, but its role in the male body is little understood.

Petrissage From the French, meaning to squeeze. The term used for any massage stroke that squeezes the muscles; for instance, kneading.

PEA (phenylethylamine) A mood-altering chemical produced in the brain and body cells. It is said to be an essential part of tender feelings, specifically 'falling in love'.

Phenylethylalcohol The 'happiness chemical' with a rose odour, related to PEA and found in chocolate, cheese, rosewater and in rose otto (the true essential oil of rose captured by steam distillation).

Pheromone A volatile substance, the subtle odour of which evokes a response in another member of the same species. Often, but not necessarily, sexual.

Resinoid Extracted from gums and resins by solvents in the same way as an absolute; for example, benzoin, a viscous extract with a vanilla-like odour.

Testosterone The male sex hormone secreted by the testes. It is also produced in the female body by the adrenal glands, but in much lower concentrations.

TMA (trimethylamine) The smell of rotting seafood. At subthreshold levels the odour is especially attractive to human males. TMA is also said to be a menstrual pheromone.

Unguent A soothing or healing salve. Also, an oil-based or fat-based perfume used in ancient times, especially in Egypt, Greece and Rome.

Volatile oil Liable to evaporation or diffusion at ordinary temperatures. Another name for an essential oil.

Bibliography

Ackerman, D. *A Natural History of the Senses* Chapmans, 1990

Annand, M. *The Art of Sexual Ecstasy*, Aquarian, 1990

Ashcroft Nowicki, D. *The Tree of Ecstacy*, Aquarian, 1991

Bahr, R. *Good Hands*, Thorsons, 1984

Burton, Sir R. *The Perfumed Garden*, Richard K. Champion, 1963

Coleman, Dr V. *Bodypower*, Thames and Hudson, 1983

Drury, N. (ed.) *Inner Health*, Prism Press, 1985

Downing, G. *The Massage Book*, Penguin, 1972

Edwards, G. *Living Magically*, Piatkus, 1991

Harrold, F. *The Massage Manual*, Headline (UK); Sterling (US); Simon & Schuster (AUS), 1992

Hendler, Dr S. *The Doctor's Vitamin and Mineral Encyclopaedia*, Arrow Books, 1991

Jellinek, Dr P. *The Practice of Modern Perfumery*, Leonard Hill, 1959

Lake, Dr M. *Scents and Sensuality*, Futura, 1989

Lawless, J. *The Encyclopaedia of Essential Oils*, Element Books, 1992

Lawrence, D. H. *Selected Stories*, Heinemann, 1976

Maury, M. *Marguerite Maury's Guide to Aromatherapy*, C.W. Daniel, 1989

O'Conner, D. *How to Make Love to the Same Person for the Rest of Your Life*, Guild Publishing, 1985

King, F. *Tantra for Westerners*, Aquarian, 1986

Kenton, L. *Ultra Health*, Ebury Press, 1984

Savill, Dr A. *Music, Health and Character*, John Lane, The Bodley Head, 1923

Sinha, I., Halu, Z. and Halu, M. *The Kama Sutra*, Thorsons, 1992

Tisserand, M. *Aromatherapy for Lovers*, Thorsons, 1993

Tisserand R. *Aromatherapy for Everyone*, Penguin, 1988

Trueman, J. *The Romantic Story of Scent*, Aldus Books, 1975

Valnet, Dr J. *The Practice of Aromatherapy*, C W. Daniel, 1980

Van Toller, S. and Dodd, G. (eds.) *Perfumer* Chapman Hall, 1988

Watson, A. and Drury, N. *Healing Music*, Prism Press, 1987

Wildwood, C. *The Aromatherapy and Massage Book*, Thorsons, 1994

Wildwood, C. *Creating Your Own Perfumes* Piatkus, 1994

Wills, P. *Colour Therapy*, Element Books, 1993

Winter, R. *The Smell Book*, J. B. Lippincott (USA), 1976

Worwood, V. A. *Aromantics*, Bantam Books, 1993

Suggested Reading

Annand, M. *The Art of Sexual Ecstasy*, Aquarian,1990

Harrold, F. *The Massage Manual*, Headline (UK); Sterling (US); Simon & Schuster (AUS), 1992

Lake, Dr M. *Scents and Sensuality*, Futura, 1989

Lawless, J. *The Encyclopaedia of Essential Oils*, Element Books, 1992

Wildwood, C. *The Aromatherapy and Massage Book*, Thorsons, 1994

Index

Acknowledgements

Many thanks, Georgina, for pointing me in the right direction, and to Judith, for your warm support of this project. Thank you so much, Chris, for the glass maiden who manifested at a significant moment – she has become a talisman of the work. I am also grateful to Paul and Marjorie Smedley of Sweet Seductions for their enthusiastic response to my request for further information on chocolate. And to my agent Susan Mears for her encouragement when the going got tough – and also to everyone at Eddison Sadd for the supportive team work. Finally, a big thank you to Rose for the imaginative Food of Love suggestions.

Eddison • Sadd Editions

Editor	Marilyn Inglis
Project Editor	Zoë Hughes
Proof Readers	Nikky Twyman
	Barbara Nash and Janet Smy
Indexer	Dorothy Frame
Art Director	Elaine Partington
Art Editor	Sarah Howerd
Bodywork Photographer	Dale Durfee
Still-life Photographer	Stephen Marwood
Production	Hazel Kirkman and
	Charles James

Eddison Sadd would like to thank the following:

The models: Debbie Flett, Andrew Markham, Regina, Darren Plull, Ralph Beck and Kay Marshall.

Prop suppliers:

Page 84 – moon and sun symbols
EQUINOX - THE ASTROLOGY SHOP
78 Neal Street, Covent Garden,
London WC2 9PA
Tel. 071 497 0344

Page 58, 82 – flowers
PAULA PRYKE
20 Penton Street,
Islington,
London N1 9PS
Tel. 071 837 7336

Pages 24, 32, 36, 40, 48, 150 – herbs/sandalwood
NEAL'S YARD REMEDIES
15 Neal's Yard,
Covent Garden,
London WC2H 9DP
Tel. 071 379 0705

Pages 24, 36, 48, 49 – botanical samples
ROYAL BOTANIC GARDENS,
Kew,
Richmond,
Surrey TW9 3AB
Tel. 081 332 5543

Chapter Openers - fabric and cushions
CHARLES & PATRICIA LESTER LTD.
Llanfoist House,
Llanfoist,
Abergavenny,
Gwent NP7 9LR

Pages 20, 30 – tables and fruit bowls
RAU
36 Islington Green,
London N1 8DU
Tel. 071 359 5337

Page 151 – square glass bottle
Page 58 – blue glass bottle
WILLIAM PRICE
25 Monmouth Street,
London WC2 H9DD
Tel. 071 379 5304
Page 77 – oil burner on left

NEW WORLD AURORA,
16a Neal's Yard,
London WC2H 9DP
Tel. 071 379 5972

Also: Charlotte Schofield, Pritty Ramjee, Karen Watts, Sarah Howerd, Hilary Krag.